NATIONAL INSTITUTE SOCIAL SERVICES LIBRARY

Volume 35

ORGANISING FOR
SOCIAL CHANGE

ORGANISING FOR SOCIAL CHANGE

A Study in the Theory and Practice of Community Work

DAVID N. THOMAS

Routledge
Taylor & Francis Group

LONDON AND NEW YORK

First published in 1976 by George Allen & Unwin Ltd

This edition first published in 2022
by Routledge
4 Park Square, Milton Park, Abingdon, Oxon OX14 4RN
605 Third Avenue, New York, NY 10017

Routledge is an imprint of the Taylor & Francis Group, an informa business

British Library Cataloguing in Publication Data
A catalogue record for this book is available from the British Library

ISBN: 978-1-03-203381-5 (Set)
ISBN: 978-1-00-321681-0 (Set) (ebk)
ISBN: 978-1-03-204286-2 (Volume 35) (hbk)
ISBN: 978-1-03-204304-3 (Volume 35) (pbk)
ISBN: 978-1-00-319136-0 (Volume 35) (ebk)

DOI: 10.4324/9781003191360

Publisher's Note
The publisher has gone to great lengths to ensure the quality of this reprint but points out that some imperfections in the original copies may be apparent.

Disclaimer
The publisher has made every effort to trace copyright holders and would welcome correspondence from those they have been unable to trace.

ORGANISING FOR SOCIAL CHANGE

A STUDY IN
THE THEORY AND PRACTICE OF COMMUNITY WORK

DAVID N. THOMAS

Lecturer in Community Work
National Institute for Social Work

With a Foreword by

PETER MARRIS

London

GEORGE ALLEN & UNWIN LTD

RUSKIN HOUSE   MUSEUM STREET

First published in 1976

© George Allen & Unwin Ltd, 1976

ISBN 0 04 361019 6

Set in 10pt Times Roman by
Linocomp Ltd, Church Street, Marcham, Oxon
Printed in Great Britain
by Biddles Ltd, Guildford, Surrey

FOREWORD

BY PETER MARRIS

This book describes an experimental intervention in a relatively poor, run-down area of Southwark by a small team of community workers. It is a sensitive account of their achievements and frustrations, and the dilemmas they faced. Its value lies not only in the experience it records, from which other community workers can learn much that is useful to their practice, but also in its evaluation of a kind of intervention, which has been increasingly resorted to as a remedy for areas with accumulating disadvantages. Educational priority areas, community development projects, inner city studies, special programmes for urban deprivation, all seek to improve the quality of life where most needed through selective, local action. These government initiatives have been matched by groups who seek through community action a handle on more radical changes. The Southwark project was neither an instrument of government, nor an expression of radical ideology, but an essentially professional initiative, and so shows particularly clearly the ambiguities of the interventionist role itself. To understand the roots of these ambiguities, we need to look back to the origins of community intervention as a strategy of reform.

After the Second World War, British social policy emphasised the national provision of services and insurance against hardship. Everyone was to be protected against poverty and misfortune, and ensured equal access to medical care, education, and decent housing as a matter of personal right. Thirty years later, this ideal is not only unrealised, but it seems more and more doubtful whether we can achieve it by a policy of universal provision for every citizen, in need or not. Again and again, economic difficulties have driven governments to cut their plans for the social services in the face of inflation and the imbalance of trade. At the same time, the complex interdependence of the economic system made government preoccupied with immediate economic regulation, at the expense of long-term plans for the redistribution of resources. Hence the disadvantaged remain dependent on means-tested relief to supplement their benefits; and their inability to find a decent home or job, or complete an adequate education, is not simply personal incompetence, to be treated by a sympathetic social worker, but a reflection of economic pressures which government cannot dominate. In these circumstances, a more selective, efficient concentration of social resources in areas of greatest need is an attractive policy. It requires only a small budget to choose a few representative deprived neighbourhoods and launch an experiment in new ways to meet their difficulties – by better co-ordination of services, encouraging self-help, innovative provisions and closer consultation with the residents themselves. On this small scale, it seems feasible to look at the situation as a whole, and master the complexity of social and economic forces which overwhelm control at national level. As in the United States, whose community action programmes inspired some British legislation, over the past ten years, appeals for a comprehensive, innovative approach to areas of special deprivation began to appear in the rhetoric of government policy, and the recommendations of committees.

At the same time, the search for more efficient management of resources has been leading, in both government and industry, to the creation of larger and larger units of organisation. Companies merged and merged again. Local government boundaries have been redrawn. The personal social services were unified on the recommendations of the Seebohm Committee. Schools grew as they became comprehensive. Departments of government have been amalgamated. Only big organisations seem able to command the resources and the breadth of attention to come to grips with the interdependence of needs and remedies. But this also makes the management of society more remote from democratic control. How are people to express their particular needs in a structure which aggregated interests into larger and larger constituencies? In its review of planning procedures, for instance, the Skeffington report began to emphasise the importance of community participation as a means of democratic control.

The frustrations which have led government towards selective local intervention also influence more radical reformers, disillusioned with conventional politics. As a means of change, political parties seem too trapped by circumstances, too hierarchical, too much the captives of powerful interests to represent effectively the needs of the poor. The Campaign for Nuclear Disarmament, the Black Power Movement in America, the student campaigns of the late sixties, and more recently the Women's Movement suggest another style of politics, more spontaneous, more aggressive, more direct – without bureaucratic structures and entrenched leadership.

If this political style is to help the poor, it too will have to begin in the streets and tenement blocks where they live.

Thus community intervention has been inspired by a search for more effective management of resources, for more effective democracy, and for a more effective means of social change. These aims merge into each other: effective management requires change and responsiveness to need; radicalism loses its momentum without democratic involvement and achievements to show. But each is distinct, and represents a different concern. Government is trying to make the most of limited resources within an economic structure that it cannot or may not wish to change radically; others see community work as a more direct attack on the way property owners or businesses threaten the interests of a neighbourhood, and a means of helping people to organise for the protection of their interests in a broader political context. The rhetoric of community action tends to disguise these different political philosophies; and despite their divergence, the immediate task may appear much the same to everyone – to help local residents articulate their needs, provide new amenities, replace or rehabilitate the worst housing, improve services and access to jobs. Thus community workers usually have to decide for themselves where their priorities lie, to whom they should ultimately be accountable, and whose interests they should sacrifice when conflicts arise.

These are political decisions. Yet community workers do not have a mandate to exercise political leadership. If they are employed by government, or – as in Southwark – by an institution, they act as professionals whose authority is limited to their vocational skills. If they are self-appointed, they are still usually outsiders whose right to intervene depends on the consent of those they are trying to help: and the justification of their claim to help is still, characteristically, the skills their education has given them. These skills are valuable: the ability to understand legislation and how local government committees work, to translate the language of bureaucracy, to organise a meeting or publicity, to keep accounts. At the same time, just because these workers devote their whole time to the common interests of the neighbourhood, they provide a secretariat with essential services – a telephone, a duplicating machine, files, a place where people can meet. But this legitimate and acknowledged role of a secretariat in practice involves an unacknowledged and questionable political intervention, however unobtrusive.

Take, for example, one of the characteristic aims of community work: to co-ordinate services so that they correspond more sensitively and efficiently with local needs. Once you invite people to express their difficulties and hardships, you undertake to help them as best you can – otherwise the invitation is dishonest. At the same time, as you report their needs to departments of local government, you discover that departments respond very differently, depending on their overall policy, and even within departments, officials are more or less sympathetic. The community worker has to become a partisan if he or she is to achieve anything – siding with this department against that, making an ally of a particular official, and prepared to become an advocate for the community against government if lobbying is unsuccessful. Similarly, if the aim is to encourage the residents of a neighbourhood to assert themselves democratically, and organise to promote their needs, it is scarcely ever possible, at the outset at least, to remain neutral about the issues to be taken up. In practice the intervener nearly always has to initiate organisation, and so has to choose the issue and the groups with whom to work most closely.

Thus community workers have to accept that their role is ambiguous. They cannot avoid making political decisions and exercising leadership, though, as professional or self-appointed helpers, they have no political mandate. And the decisions they take will be influenced by their interpretation of the ambiguous aims of community action itself. Forced to choose, should they sacrifice their commitment to local democracy for the sake of helping local government put through a policy for more effective management? Or sacrifice official co-operation by whole-hearted advocacy of the community point of view? Or pursue a conflict uncompromisingly so as to raise people's awareness of the need for more radical changes? What matters most – better government, more democratic involvement, more revolutionary consciousness? The choice cannot be derived from the formal terms of employment, but only from the personal philosophy which guides one's sense of responsibility. The choices are never comfortable, and the point at which one has to choose is seldom obvious: when does compromise become co-optation? When is the unwillingness to compromise stultifying? In the end, these questions lead back to the ambiguity inherent in the origins of community action. It was provoked by the frustrations of national policy: yet local intervention cannot easily influence national issues.

Poverty, unemployment and bad housing may be concentrated in particular neighbourhoods, but their causes are seldom local. Hence community action is continually frustrated by its inability to come to grips with the remoter, underlying sources of the disadvantages it is trying to tackle. It cannot substitute for national policies to relieve unemployment, finance cheap housing, or provide services. It has to be conceived as complementing or stimulating such policies. So, for instance, an experiment in co-ordinating services and making them more sensitive to need is a dishonest evasion of the problems if resources are not then provided either to meet the needs which come to light or to implement the findings of the experiment elsewhere. Even if a community worker is concerned primarily with the well-being of the residents in one neighbourhood, he or she has to take account of the relevance of that work to the major factors which influence their welfare. This is the context in which a worker has finally to decide whether it is more useful to improve the competence of local government, enable people to organise, or raise their awareness of the roots of their problems. Sooner or later, the pursuit of one of these aims will alienate allies who might help pursue the others.

In practice, these issues seldom present themselves cleanly, when they might be decided on principle, but more as continual doubts and dilemmas. The achievements of community work are always caught in a double bind. Every success raises the question: did it buy off the challenge to undertake less superficial remedies? Every failure confirms the impotence of ordinary people to assert their interests.

This study does not attempt to resolve these ambiguities, or to reach a conclusive evaluation of the Southwark experiment. It provides a searching, self-critical account of several years' experience, which shows how one team struggled with the issues as they evolved. It offers, too, a framework for assessing the achievements, which avoids both tautological pessimism and complacency, but asks the testing question. Readers must decide for themselves whether the experiment justified the cost; whether the team chose the right priorities and the most appropriate role. But the project did help to foster local organisations of continuing vitality, and it influenced the solution to some of the most urgent housing needs. The study shows the rewards, as well as the doubts and frustrations, of a kind of intervention whose power to help deserves to be continually discriminated, explored and developed.

PREFACE

This book attempts to describe the different stages in the process of community work and to delineate the tasks, roles and skills of community workers. It is also an attempt to conceptualise the community work process and the relationship of community work interventions to the issues which currently occupy the attention of neighbourhood groups. Finally, the book is about the work of the Southwark Community Project undertaken by the National Institute for Social Work. Field records and other reports from this Project provide the raw materials for the description and analysis of community work practice.

National Institute staff and students who participated in the Southwark Community Project as well as staff from other agencies and local residents will doubtless recognise some of their own thinking in this book. However, although many people's ideas have contributed to the making of this book, responsibility for the opinions and ideas expressed is the author's and they do not necessarily represent those of the National Institute for Social Work nor those of other community workers who have been on the staff of the Southwark Community Project.

ACKNOWLEDGEMENTS

This book owes most of its inspiration to the prodigious efforts of local people in north-west Southwark to achieve changes in and for their neighbourhood. Many ideas evolved as a result of the interaction between Project workers, community groups and statutory and voluntary agencies in Southwark; in describing community action in north-west Southwark we may have done less than justice to the overall work and policies of these agencies.

Many people have contributed to the shape and content of the book. Dorothy Runnicles wrote Chapter 8 and provided material for Chapters 2, 3 and 9. Her advice and comments on the whole of the book proved invaluable. Use has been made of the field records and papers written at different times of Elizabeth Radford, Dorothy Runnicles, David Thomas, Harley Frank, Jef Smith, Naomi Honigsbaum, John Harding, Joan Ballentine, John Rea Price, Jeremy Burnett, John Austin and Dick Ehlers.

The Southwark Community Project's Advisory Committee supported and encouraged the work in north-west Southwark and members read and commented upon early and final drafts. Peter Marris and David Jones also undertook detailed reading. The main burden of critical and creative editing was undertaken by Professor Harry Specht, on a year's leave at the National Institute for Social Work from his duties in the School of Social Welfare at Berkeley, California. He not only helped in the editing of the book but also in the development of the thoughts and ideas that went into its making.

David Jones was responsible, as Director of the Project, for an immense amount of skilled and devoted work with Project staff. The depth and significance of his work are barely captured in the text of the book, and the opportunity is taken here to acknowledge his contribution to the work of the Project and the personal and professional development of its workers.

Finance for the Southwark Community Project was provided by the City Parochial Foundation, the Goldsmiths Company and the Joseph Rowntree Charitable Trust, whose generous support far exceeded the original estimates for this Project and whose interest and support are gratefully acknowledged.

Several staff members at the National Institute, particularly Catherine Briscoe, helped to lighten the teaching load of the author so that he could work on completing the book.

Thanks are also due to those who helped to prepare the manuscript – Jean Sheldrake, Penny Fouche, Paddy Field, Bernadette Springer, Doris Kent, Maggie Dunne, Ellen McKenna, Rosina Shaw and Priscilla Foley.

Finally, thanks to Oula Jones who, under exacting circumstances, 'writes indexes to perfection'.

CONTENTS

INTRODUCTION

From its inception in 1961 the National Institute for Social Work had been concerned with what was originally referred to as 'training for social work with communities'. Its concern to provide training facilities in this field was supported by a series of reports through the middle 1960s.[1] The need for community work at that time was argued against the background of the shift away from institutions to community care, and the need to augment the personal social services in deprived inner city neighbourhoods. It was also viewed as a means of meeting the social problems of deteriorating neighbourhoods, and of special groups within the community. Finally, with one eye on the alleged political apathy and disenchantment of the British voter, there was the need to 'strengthen the democratic process . . . by enabling people to articulate their needs to decide what they want for their communities and to bring this about by their own efforts'.[2]

But in 1967 the National Institute found that there were few experienced community work practitioners and little opportunity for students to gain the practical experience essential for training. The Institute therefore proposed a field project in the London area where community work skills could be developed with workers sufficiently experienced to undertake the required teaching.

The Institute appointed three field staff and located the project in the London Borough of Southwark which was easily accessible from the Institute. In addition, several voluntary and local authority agencies had expressed their eagerness to co-operate with the project. The Institute had contacts with many agencies in Southwark and it also had a major research project under way involving work with the welfare and health departments in the borough.

---

[1] *Social Work and the Community. Proposals for Reorganising Local Authority Services in Scotland* (HMSO, 1966); *The Needs of New Communities* (HMSO, 1967); *Children and their Primary Schools*, 2 vols (HMSO, 1966); A. Leissner, *Family Advice Services* (Longmans, London 1967); *Community Work and Social Change*, Calouste Gulbenkian Foundation (Longmans, London 1968).

[2] *Proposal for a Project on Social Work with Communities* (NISW, 1967), p. 1.

The first staff appointment to the Southwark Community Project (SCP) was made in 1968, and the team moved into Southwark later in the same year. Work in north-west Southwark started in January 1969, and continued for some three and a half years, during which time slums were pulled down and people rehoused, playgrounds were opened, plans successfully challenged and opposed, issues taken up and explored, gardens opened and libraries perpetuated, councillors and officers persuaded and pressured, and service agencies pushed and pulled towards a better understanding of the welfare of those in the community most in need of care and respect.

The vortex of the Project's activity, and that of most of the neighbourhood groups who used its resources, comprised the struggle to achieve improvements in the housing of those who lived in the slums that dominated many parts of north-west Southwark. The Project worked with some thirteen tenants' associations, most of whom sought rehousing for their members, some of whom were striving for modernisation of their accommodation and for improvements in recreational and maintenance facilities. The sites of demolished slums have been taken over by the children, eager to colonise any land that will augment the impoverished play provision of the area. In addition, two groups of local residents secured derelict sites for adventure playgrounds, staffed and equipped them and obtained long-term financing through Urban Aid and the Inner London Education Authority.

Housing and play provision were the twin pivots in the Project's neighbourhood work. But Project staff also worked with groups concerned with a range of local, regional and, in some cases, national issues. The following were primary amongst the issues that, together with housing and play, took up the interest and time of its neighbourhood workers: redevelopment of the riverside, the level of health care, community newspapers, the early detection and prevention of homelessness, the preservation of local gardens and the library, pedestrian-crossing provision, parent–teacher associations, support for flat-bound mothers, welfare rights, the level of employment opportunities, and the erosion of shopping and transport facilities.

Work with community groups entailed continuing contact with staff in the statutory and voluntary services. One Project team member was given responsibility for working with service agencies with the objectives of aiding community orientation of individual services and of promoting inter-agency planning and approaches to community needs. A number of collaborative assignments were undertaken by the Project with agency staff and some of this work has been published.[1]

The activities of the Project and neighbourhood groups and their interaction with service agencies did not take place in a social and political vacuum. The work of the Project, which in 1968 was amongst the first major attempts at community work intervention in Great Britain, influenced and was influenced by a number of other variables that locally and nationally determined the climate in which neighbourhood groups could be successful in achieving some measure of social change. The work of the SCP, and that of the groups and service agencies, was conditioned by the wide variety of commitments to community action that, under a diversity of names, flourished in the late '60s and early '70s. Not even the most entrenched and paternalistic of local authorities could escape from acknowledging the consequences of the sanctions that were being given to community action by the plethora of reports (e.g. Seebohm, Skeffington, Gulbenkian) and national programmes (e.g. Urban Aid, the Community Development Projects) that, explicitly or by implication, praised the virtues of self-help and participation and called for greater responsiveness of service providers to community need.

Community action on local needs quickly became a component of political life in town halls in urban communities. Councillors and officers who chose to reflect that the government of their borough would 'not be influenced by pressure groups' were disabused of these notions by the activities of the squatting movement which helped to alert residents to the possibilities of collective action on local needs and grievances. At the same time, there was a transformation of the efforts of students and other activists who had spent their non-working hours in helping the deprived, whether homeless families, gypsies or rent-striking council tenants. This transformation took the form of the professionalisation of the skills and contribution of these committed and knowledgeable strangers who identified with, and organised around, the needs of residents in deprived urban neighbourhoods. The Association of Community Workers was inaugurated in the autumn of 1968, and there was a steady increase in the number of educational institu-

[1] See Appendix B for a list of SCP publications.

tions that made some provision for teaching in community work. Major trusts and charities were soon to notice the increasing numbers of applications that came to them from churches, councils of social service, teaching institutions, and indigenous groups concerned with a variety of issues, all seeking funds for some kind of community organising, often employing a full-time field worker. These were some of the features of the changing climate in which the Southwark Community Project (SCP) developed in the years between 1968 and 1973.

A paradox of the Project's work is that it contributed to the break-up of a community and the erosion of its identity through the success of demolishing slums whose inhabitants were dispersed throughout the borough. Yet those very successes in slum demolition were an integral part of a more general movement which served to strengthen the cohesion and identity of the community. Because of the cumulative success in collective action, and because of the work of one local group in stressing the needs of the total neighbourhood in the physical reshaping of the area, the interests and views of residents of north-west Southwark, whether as a neighbourhood or as members of disparate groups around local issues, can no longer be neglected with impunity. 'There is', as one councillor remarked, 'a voice in the north.' The Southwark Community Project, along with other agencies and individuals, helped to organise and support that voice.

It is more sobering to reflect that the Project could do little to help those individuals and families who were living out their days in poverty. Some joined in collective action on neighbourhood issues but few were deceived into thinking that their escape from poverty could be achieved only, if at all, through highly localised community action. Community work operates on the margins of those national economic forces that oppress many working-class families in this country. Within these margins, there is much that can be achieved on the local level, even though we can speculate that many resources (e.g. new housing chances, playgrounds) which came to north-west Southwark were probably diverted from, and at the expense of, residents living in other equally deprived situations in Southwark or Inner London. This is, surely, one of the most interesting and complex issues that confronts community work. However, while it is one of which the Project workers were conscious, their activities concerned one locality and only occasionally extended to some of these larger city-wide and national issues.

We move, then, to the first chapter, where the Project is described as one of many interacting resources in the area. We discuss the notion of the relevance of any particular resource to the neighbourhood in which it is based. Measures are put forward for assessing relevance and we encourage the reader to apply them to the work of the Project as it is revealed in subsequent pages.

Chapter 1

THE RELEVANCE AND VALUE OF NEIGHBOURHOOD RESOURCES

In this chapter we provide some criteria for assessing the contribution of the SCP as a *resource* to the community in north-west Southwark. To do this we indicate briefly the kinds of needs to which the Project's resources were thought to be relevant. We then present in the final section of the chapter a more general framework within which most kinds of community resources (for instance, social services, housing and employment opportunities) can be measured for the contribution they make to meeting the needs of people living in the kind of deprived inner-city neighbourhood described in this book.

We have chosen to emphasise the notion of 'community resources' for two major reasons. First, much that is practised and written about in that strand of community work concerned with direct work with local people assumes that the alliance of professional and community group can influence resources at a local level. Residents are encouraged to identify and articulate their needs and take collective action in respect of them. That action is mostly about influencing decision-makers in the way they allocate resources to groups or neighbourhoods. More importantly, collective action is seen as the means through which local residents develop skills and confidence to improve the contribution they make as *human* resources to the process of decision-making about *material* resources in and on behalf of their neighbourhood.

Second, it is necessary (if community work is partly or mainly about influencing local resources) to be able to measure the contribution of a resource to meeting needs in a neighbourhood; and further, to measure changes in a resource's capacity to meet needs as a consequence of action taken by local residents. We do not pretend in this chapter to present a means of measurement that is wholly adequate. We have only attempted to suggest a way of looking at community resources that will help readers to be more exact about the effects of one kind of community resource as it intervened in the lives of local residents in one part of London.

THE 'RELEVANCE' OF COMMUNITY RESOURCES

In considering the Southwark Community Project (SCP) as a 'community resource' a good starting point is to consider the notion of 'relevance'. If we assume an intended correspondence between resources and the needs of a local community, then the 'relevance' of that resource depends on several factors, including:

the location of that resource within or reasonably near to the community with which it is concerned;
the way in which the resource is presented to consumer groups;
the identification of the resource workers with the needs of people in a neighbourhood;
the extent of participation of resource users in planning and making policy decisions about the resource.

There are, of course, many other factors but these are particularly important for a community work project that is seeking to establish its relevance within a local community. The SCP, like many other similar operations, was an externally motivated, planned and financed intervention. There was no survey of local opinion when the team members decided to open up a neighbourhood base. The Project was not invited in by local residents and groups. Nor had the voluntary and statutory agencies, many of whom had welcomed the appearance of the Project, envisaged that it would move into a neighbourhood and strengthen the residents vis-à-vis those very same agencies. But in 1968, community work projects were comparatively untried ventures both for local residents and service agencies. Even today, despite the enormous growth of community action, the level of understanding of community work projects is low compared with people's understanding of other resources like the Department of Health and Social Security and the local 'welfare' offices. The local community in 1968 had no available experience or local institution to which they could compare the appearance and activities of the Project and its workers. In these circumstances it was vital that care was taken in the way the Project and its workers were presented to potential users.

One set of users were the service agencies in the borough. The first worker to be appointed spent several months in Southwark defining the possible roles for the Project and gathering the expectations of the various services. We find that the Project was described in some of the following ways: a neighbourhood project was wanted 'in probably a high pathological area which was fairly defined geographically'; to help Southwark 'to develop an increased sense of community relevance in its activities as a result of Project efforts'; the object of the Project was 'to influence and change perspectives of the widest range of people in the borough so that they become more and more community minded'. The team member responsible for developing work with the service agencies described the Project staff as 'interested in helping individuals and groups with problems and issues relating to their service in the area which were of concern and priority, and in collecting and sharing information and views about the nature of local problems to which an agency might be able to make a relevant contribution'.

The other set of consumers was, of course, the residents of that part of the borough to which the Project would direct its resources. In January 1969, the Project team decided to work in the London Bridge area. The decision was taken after a series of constituency ward studies which indicated that this area contained some of the most deprived neighbourhoods in Southwark. The Project started to establish its relevance to the needs of that area by moving into it. The move to a local base represented a parochialisation of Project resources in respect of work with neighbourhood groups. Although the Project workers operated on a borough-wide basis on social planning issues, they seldom undertook work with neighbourhood groups outside the target area. Identification with a specific neighbourhood also gave the Project a constituency which helped to validate the Project's work with service agencies. However, as the Project became more useful and relevant to local groups, many of whom were in conflict with the local authority, the agencies found the Project a less acceptable resource with which to collaborate. The Project developed as a resource within and relevant to a specific north-west Southwark neighbourhood and accepted the constraints that this placed on opportunities to work with agencies and neighbourhood interests from other parts of Southwark.

The decision to locate the Project in the London Bridge area implied that the team saw a correspondence between the Project's resources and needs in the neighbourhood. This is not to say that the Project was adequate as a resource, because the team were always aware of work not being followed through or taken up, or adequately covered by the two or three workers available. Project resources could not meet all the needs in the locality. But there was some expectation that the resources, even if they were insufficient, were appropriate to the needs of the local community. But these resources were such that they could not meet the *material* needs of the residents in the locality. The Project was not in business to meet these kinds of needs, nor to persuade people who did provide resources, such as housing, to make them available to individuals and families in the area. Rather, the resources of the Project corresponded with the *organisational needs* of local people – the need for advice and encouragement in articulating material needs and objectives, and taking collective action in respect of them.

This distinction between material and organisational needs is useful if only to stave off the sense of futility that overtakes many community workers in their daily work. This sense of futility is bred by the inextricable knit of national policies with local problems and resources. The SCP never argued that, by acting in a local area, the difficulties and problems that were faced by the residents of that neighbourhood could be removed. What the Project team came to recognise more forcibly during their work was that no local effort by residents alone, or with whatever paid help is available, can change the total environment of the people who live in a deprived neighbourhood.

There are, however, a variety of reasons why individuals continue as community workers even when they recognise some of the extreme limitations of their work. For some it is the knowledge that whatever structural change occurs nationally to the economic system it will not be possible to win and perpetuate such changes unless residents of deprived neighbourhoods have become more confident and more skilled in taking hold of any redistribution of resources and the power and opportunities that come from holding them. There is also the belief that more extensive structural change will not occur only because of desire and commitment but must be worked towards in ways that are sometimes very small. The assertion by community groups of purely parochial interests may lead them to a better understanding of the inadequacies of economic systems responsible for the creation and perpetuation of areas of social deprivation.

The function of a resource like the SCP in meeting the organisational needs of a community, in preparing people to take hold of the opportunities that more extensive structural change may bring, is crucial. The schools, valiant though the efforts of some teachers are, cannot compensate for the children's early years in a slum. Instead they often produce for the child from a deprived area like north-west Southwark a series of events than confirm his view that he, and those who share his experiences, are failures. In these circumstances, a resource like the SCP which is concerned with the organisational needs of communities is a force for community education. It is not the only force, for the Project found that some of the men who took active roles in community action had acquired and developed their organisational skills within the trade union movement.

ORGANISATIONAL NEEDS AND SKILLS

In order to influence decisions about the use and distribution of resources in such a way as to optimise their contribution to the wellbeing of the neighbourhood, local people and groups must first begin to *identify* those whom the electorate or education or sheer good luck have marked out as the decision-makers in respect of community resources. Here we refer to local authority councillors and officers, private landlords, businessmen, teachers, doctors, social workers and other professionals and administrators including those in central government. Having identified those decision-makers (who, of course, change with disconcerting frequency) and the resources for which they are responsible, local people must also decide on the *unit of organisation* that will be used to press the community interest. People might decide to relate individually or collectively to decision-makers. If collectively, as was invariably the case in north-west Southwark, there are always a number of forms of organisation that have to be considered and tested out. Once this unit of organisation is selected, residents must simultaneously develop their own skills and resources as a group and *negotiate* with the decision-makers about the resource in question whether it be a plot of land that might be used for a playground or a compulsory purchase order for a slum. Both tasks involve acquiring or augmenting skills and vocabularies such as how to run a committee, recruit new members, talk to the Press, use the telephone, write letters, organise petitions and deputations, arrange demonstrations, negotiate for funds and, with some resources such as a playground, employ staff. All these jobs require skills that will enable individuals and groups to influence, for the interests of their constituents, decisions about neighbourhood resources. The tasks of identification, organisation, self-development and negotiation precipitate local people towards the acquisition and growth of organisational skills, and this was a practical need to which the staff of the SCP was ready to respond.

TYPES OF COMMUNITY RESOURCES

The growth of organisational skills takes place within the context of improving the well-being of the neighbourhood and specific groups within it. It is possible to characterise an area like north-west Southwark in terms of the stock and variety of neighbourhood resources that are relevant to the overall well-being of residents. There appear to be four broad categories of resources, though there is considerable overlap among them. First, there exists what might be called the *material resources* of a neighbourhood. These primarily are the existing housing stock, the quantity and range of job opportunities in the area (recognising, of course, that many men travel outside north-west Southwark for work), the number, type and quality of schools, the amount and kind of open space, the neighbourhood's transport systems and, finally, the present use and zoning of the stock of land in the neighbourhood.

The second category we refer to as *commercial service resources*, and we would include here the neighbourhood's shops, clubs, pubs, theatres and cinemas.

The third category comprises the *organisational support resources* in the neighbourhood. This includes the churches, local settlements, the local authority's social service department, the local offices of the Department of Health and Social Security, local councillors, and professionals like doctors and health visitors.

The fourth and last category includes the stock of emotional and intellectual resources of fortitude and resilience within persons and families, the wage-earning capacities of wives and elder children, the network of local friends and relatives and the closeness and familiarity of these neighbourhood ties, and the networks through which families acquire material resources cheaply, either legitimately or criminally. These resources we call *internal support resources* because they are relevant to people in their day-to-day life, particularly when they need support because of a temporary or continuing inability or unwillingness to obtain sufficient material and/or organisational support resources.

The relationship between each of these resources is dynamic and constantly changing. If we were to portray this relationship schematically we would obtain some understanding of the links in the social network that binds inhabitants of neighbourhoods like north-west Southwark. Failure to achieve within the educational system is related to inadequate opportunities for housing and employment. Families caught in this circle will rely on organisational and internal support resources to sustain daily life. The social security office may provide supplementary benefits or a family income supplement; the area social workers and the church may provide support to families in stress caused or aggravated by bad housing and low income; the doctor and health visitor will help to repair or prevent damages to health caused by bad housing and an unbalanced diet; the local councillor may press a family's claim for better accommodation. Wives and elder children will work to augment the low income of husbands, and families will exploit, and be exploited by, the retailers of cheap or stolen commodities. The strength to survive in these circumstances might come from neighbourhood friends and relatives as well as from an internal supply of fortitude and resignation.

These neighbourhood resources correspond, with varying degrees of fit, to the needs and problems of people and groups in the community. The SCP was concerned to improve this fit and to this end adopted two major strategies. The first was to work with service agencies in the borough to help them become more aware of and responsive to neighbourhood needs and priorities. The second strategy was to work with local people at the level of their organisational needs to enable them to exert more control and influence over the way in which resources were used and distributed within their community. There are at least two assumptions behind both strategies. The first is that agencies and individuals who controlled and allocated resources did not do so in ways that contributed optimally to meeting needs in north-west Southwark. Here we refer to the way in which resources were distributed within the borough as a whole and to the manner in which they were used once they had been allocated to meeting needs in north-west

Southwark. This assumption involves the key questions about participation and accountability in resource control and allocation: Who has the decision-making powers in respect of a resource? Does the community to whom a resource is relevant have any responsibility for, or participation in, decisions made about the resources? What gives resource decision-makers their status? That is, to whom are they accountable for their decisions about neighbourhood resources? Are they democratically elected councillors or land developers with a major responsibility to their shareholders?

The second assumption is that the search for, and attainment of, community influence in decision-making about resources helps to achieve the fit between those resources and the community needs to which they are *intended* to be relevant; or to which they have *ceased* to be relevant and consequently aggravate, as in the case of slum housing; or to which they are *potentially* relevant, as in the case of derelict land that could be used to provide open space facilities.

The question of the fit between general resources and parochial needs is concerned with what we shall call the *value of a community resource*. Any resource may be said to have one or more of three values: *financial*, *social*, and *neighbourhood*. A school, for instance, has a financial value and a social value to the extent that it carries out its educational functions. Its neighbourhood value can be assessed by the degree to which it is designed to meet, and actually succeeds in meeting, the educational needs of the community in which it is situated. It would be very difficult, for instance, to assign much neighbourhood value to a private fee-paying school that is situated in a deprived neighbourhood. Not only would such a resource be indifferent to the educational needs of that community but it would carry a high opportunity cost since the land might justifiably be used for a resource like a state school or council housing which could make a real contribution to meeting some of the community's needs.

Thus we can say that the quest for influence over the use and disposal of resources is also a quest to optimise the value of a resource to a particular neighbourhood. There are several criteria by which we can measure or assess the neighbourhood value of resources found in deprived inner-city neighbourhoods. In the first place we can ask: does the resource adequately meet the needs of the local population; does it adequately respond to the demands made upon it by its actual or potential users? Asking the question in this second way enables us to see that many resources have such a limited neighbourhood value that they actually inhibit demands made upon them by community users and hence aggravate the limitations of their value. An example of such a resource would be an out-of-touch service agency that attracts little use; or a slum block which has so deteriorated that it attracts users who normally have very little choice on the housing market such as tramps and alcoholics whose presence makes the building even less attractive for other groups in the community in housing need. It can be argued, of course, that any one of the slums in north-west Southwark had some neighbourhood value. Such a building provided centre-city housing near to a man's place of work at a very low rent. Any roof is better than no roof. There may have been some categories of tenants whose housing needs were adequately met by a slum, and there may be a clash here between the demands made upon a slum by some of its tenants and the expectations of society at large (and many slum dwellers) about the kind of housing provision appropriate to Britain in the 1970s.

The second measure of neighbourhood value is whether the use of a resource will bring other resources into use in the neighbourhood. For instance, when a plot of waste land is converted into a resource of neighbourhood value like an adventure playground, other resources are attracted to the area in the form of playleaders, volunteer helpers, children's outings, and football tournaments. At the same time, the use of the playground may lead to a reduction in the use of other resources like the police and the educational welfare and probation services; it may also lead to an increase in the use of a neighbouring resource like a local swimming pool or library. We shall consider this a *positive* redistribution of resource use, and we can assign considerable neighbourhood value to a resource that promotes such a redistribution. On the other hand some resources will lead to a *negative* redistribution of resource use. For instance, the perpetuation of a slum will lead to the diversion of a whole battery of other, quite expensive, resources. Social workers, public health inspectors, doctors and health visitors are some of the resources that will be deployed to help with the problems caused by, or associated with, bad housing. Thus the second measure is: does the resource lead to a positive or negative redistribution of resource use? This is a complex measurement. One can, for instance, imagine a situation where most of the resources brought in to cope with the consequences of bad housing conditions (e.g. social workers, doctors) might collaborate with a tenants' movement and prove to be instrumental in getting the slum cleared and demolished. The deployment of these organisational support resources is negative (if only for their high opportunity cost) and confirms the low neighbourhood value of the slum to the extent that these support resources continue to give only casework help and advice to individual families and by so doing help to perpetuate the existence of a low-value resource. This perpetuation is achieved because casework may help individual families to get out of a slum but their accommodation becomes available for other families. When these support resources provide, in addition to casework help, social change assistance such as collaboration with tenants to demolish a slum, the collaboration and the demolition both confirm the slum's low neighbourhood value and enhance the value of those organisational support resources to the community.

Our third measure of the neighbourhood value of a resource is whether its existence enhances or diminishes the neighbourhood value of other resources. For example a slum may devalue the functioning of resources like the local schools because children's housing conditions prevent them from making the most of the school's educational opportunities. Here, for instance, is how a Project worker reported a headmaster's description of the effect on his school of a local slum building:

'Mr Hodson said that most of the accommodation of the children meant that there was mixed teenage sleeping in the majority of the families and many of the younger children couldn't get off to bed because they had to sleep in the living room. The school had constantly noticed that many of the children were too tired to work at school; their attainment was low and their vocabulary stunted and he put this down to some large extent to lack of sleep. He said that it quite often happens that children are very tired for quite a period of time and then have a few days off school; he thinks that this is to catch up on sleep.

'The accommodation means that there is no place to store playthings and there are no adequate play facilities in the neighbourhood. They noticed for instance that many of the girls spend a lot of time "tidying up" and they find that, in their lessons, numbers of girls in each class seem to get most satisfaction not out of playing or learning but from the tidying-up process.

'They have stopped homework since seeing the accommodation that families had to manage in during the recent teachers'

strike and feel that because children have nowhere to do homework it really is inappropriate to set it.'

The fourth measure is whether the perpetuation of a resource
precludes the introduction of more benign or more harmful resources. If we refer again to the slum, we must make an assessment
of neighbourhood value that takes into account what would be put
on the site if it were demolished. The slum's low neighbourhood
value would be enhanced if we found that its perpetuation was
holding back the extension of a school or the redevelopment of the
land for new housing. If the site were earmarked for office development or heavy lorry parking facilities, the community might consider this being of less neighbourhood value than school or housing
development. Another example is a resource like a power station
or chemical plant whose operations make the adjoining land un-
suitable for housing or open space. Although such a use would
have some neighbourhood value (e.g. jobs), this must be balanced
against the fact that its presence precludes the creation of resources
with a high neighbourhood value such as housing.

We are not saying that every resource must be assessed only by
its contribution to the neighbourhood in which it is sited. Every
neighbourhood has to accommodate some resource whose contribution is perhaps to the region or to the city as a whole. We
recognise, for instance, that the outer suburbs of London must take
their share of council housing and accept more responsibility for
homeless families in the inner city even though they may feel such
provision has little or no neighbourhood value. We are here talking
about areas like north-west Southwark which are already severely
deprived and we believe that such areas already have more than
their share of low-value resources and may have to welcome many
more. Motorway schemes and the demolition of flats and shops to
make way for office development and uncongenial industrial uses
more often take place in areas that are less able to oppose their
introduction and that have every reason to demand the introduction of high-value resources like public housing, schools and open
space.

The four measures of neighbourhood value that have been put
forward in this chapter are implicit in the description and evaluation of the work of the Southwark Community Project. In the next
chapter we describe the neighbourhood resources as they were
found at the beginning of the Project's work. An account is then

given of how the Project workers[1] and local groups interacted with these resources in an attempt to change their value to the northwest Southwark neighbourhood. The Project was an organisational support resource whose staff worked with other neighbourhood resources (e.g. service agencies and local groups) to achieve changes in the material resources of the area as well as changes in the servicedelivery patterns of agencies and community groups. On occasions, the Project became a temporary part of the internal support network of the neighbourhood.

[1] The term 'workers' is used in the text to include not only staff members but also the many students on placement at the SCP.

Chapter 2

CRITERIA FOR INTERVENTION: NEEDS AND RESOURCES IN INNER CITY AREAS

Attempts within urban communities to effect social change through community work interventions have been focused almost exclusively upon inner city neighbourhoods with certain types of characteristics. These neighbourhoods, frequently referred to as 'areas of multiple deprivation', are often characterised by most or all of the following problems: bad housing, poor school facilities, poverty and unemployment, a deteriorating environment, inadequate play provision, unreliable transport and communications systems and the inadequate provision and take-up of organisational support services.

Urban communities have many such neighbourhoods and community workers will be faced with the task of choosing a neighbourhood in which to locate the resources of a community work project. In this chapter we describe the neighbourhood in which the Southwark Community Project was based and the kinds of resources that Project workers found in north-west Southwark. We outline the area's history and environment, and the resources available for providing residents with homes and jobs, remembering that a description of a resource may also be a description of the needs of the people within that community. The chapter ends with a profile of some of the organisational support services.

SELECTING A TARGET AREA

The London Borough of Southwark was formed in April 1965 from the old Metropolitan boroughs of Southwark, Bermondsey and Camberwell. It has a population of approximately 300,000 and it stretches from the Thames in the north to Crystal Palace in the south. Bermondsey, Rotherhithe, the Borough, the Elephant and Castle, Camberwell, Peckham and Dulwich are the familiar names of some of its communities, which are quite different from one another in terms of their character, housing, social amenities and community problems.

Within north-west Southwark, the Project adopted as its target area the borough district which was the unit used by the Planning Department for its proposed structure plans. This area of some 32,870 persons is encompassed within a square mile, bordered on the north by the River Thames from the borough boundary (which runs almost parallel with Blackfriars Road) to Tower Bridge on the east, dropping south to the New Kent Road and along to the Elephant and Castle, and there north again behind the Imperial War Museum. The target area comprised two complete wards and fragments of two others. The SCP ward study was carried out in Cathedral Ward.

The boundaries of these wards and of the planning district did not define the boundaries of the neighbourhoods to which people *felt* they belonged. These neighbourhoods were much smaller units and were determined by factors like place and type of residence, place of work and by shopping and recreational patterns. Local residents in this area often referred to themselves as living in the Borough, whilst others would refer to the Elephant, or to Bermondsey or to Bankside as the neighbourhood to which they were attached and by which they wished to be known. With the exception of two estates near the Elephant and Castle, most of the work of the Project was carried out within and on the borders of Cathedral Ward. The neighbourhood groups that used the Project were, with two exceptions, resident within a quarter of a mile of the Project premises, and the catchment area for work with individual families and persons who came for information and advice was usually much smaller – less than 200 yards from the Project door.

THE COMMUNITY'S HISTORICAL HERITAGE

Hundreds of tourists come each year to north-west Southwark, attracted by the Cathedral and the neighbourhood's association with Shakespeare and Dickens. The visitors drink beer in riverside pubs close to the spot where Chaucer's pilgrims set off for Canterbury. The neighbourhood's history is a resource of which local residents are proud; yet, sometimes ambivalence sets in during the summer season when the streets and pubs are congested with tourists, taxing diminishing shopping and catering services which add insult to injury by putting up prices in order to capture more of the tourist revenue. This revenue is not channelled back into the community whose history seems more important than its present needs and problems. Of course, local shops, pubs and breweries benefit from this resource, but the shops are owned either by larger retail units or by small and middle-sized entrepreneurs who take their profits home with them to the outer suburbs.

The history of Cathedral Ward and the adjacent ward of Riverside is the early history of Southwark. The area is immediately opposite to the City of London, and it provided, until the middle of the eighteenth century, the only crossing point to the north side of the river. The settlement that developed around London Bridge has been urban since Roman times, whilst much of the remaining area in north-west Southwark was rural until the mid-nineteenth century. Not only did London Bridge's role as the only passing point over to the City endow the south bank with a communication or corridor role (which is responsible for much of the appearance of the area today), but north-west Southwark developed as a vital source of services, labour and supplies to the City of London. There was rapid population growth in the first half of the nineteenth century, with the population doubling between 1801 and 1851. Urbanisation developed rapidly and the area became what Pevsner has described as 'a very unwholesome mixture of slums and towering warehouses cut across in all directions by railway viaducts and bridges'. By 1851, Cathedral Ward had been completely covered by development and the area grew rapidly as a mixed residential, industrial and wharf-warehousing centre servicing the rest of the city.

THE ENVIRONMENT

The residents of north-west Southwark live in an environment that is still chiefly determined by features of the historical development of the area outlined in the preceding section. Wherever one walks in the area, one is conscious of its importance as a corridor, funnelling traffic down on to three road bridges and two railway bridges.

The railway line from London Bridge to Waterloo divides the area into two sections. Residential development to the north of this line is limited and extremely isolated. The river frontage and its immediate hinterland is given over to wharves and warehouses. This is an area with an atmosphere all of its own – the stark blackness of towering, Victorian warehouses interspersed with narrow alleys that lead into the riverside and which, at low tide, permit access to the foreshore and remarkable views of the river and City. There is the occasional pub and eighteenth-century house that bears witness to the life of the past, as do the plaques that mention the different theatres. The line of warehouses and cranes is broken by the hugh Bankside power station which belches soot and smoke over the area during the day. Near the power station are the modern complexes of central government buildings including offices of the Department of the Environment and the Ministry of Defence. The way in which central government and commercial enterprises are overflowing into north-west Southwark indicates a new use by the city of its southern hinterland.

But residential dwellings account for about half the southern section of the area, and relatively less land is given over to commerce and industry. There are four schools, a local children's hospital, and several corner shops, but the noise, dirt and traffic unrelieved by green space or trees and overshadowed by the railway arches, contribute to the unmitigated drabness of the area. Open space was a particular problem in both the northern and southern sections of the area in which the Project worked. Indeed, the entire London Borough of Southwark had an open space deficiency of some 300 acres. The public open space that existed in the Project area was poor and under-equipped, usually bare, tarred playgrounds set amongst warehouses and industrial land.

The target area of the SCP was environmentally deprived, combining drab and dirty land uses with some of the worst service and recreational facilities in the whole of the borough. The environment consisted of traffic systems and redundant resources which oppressed the area with their bleakness. Decaying warehouses and industrial premises have a considerable opportunity cost in an area that is in great need of resources with a high neighbourhood value like housing, jobs and open space. The environmental deficiencies of the neighbourhood when the Project came to the area were compounded by a virtual planning blight, as the two planning authorities (the London Borough of Southwark and the Greater London Council) prepared their respective development plans for the riverside and its hinterland.

DEMOGRAPHIC CHARACTERISTICS OF RESIDENTS

North-west Southwark is a predominantly working-class neighbourhood. Of the neighbourhood's occupied and retired men, some 40 per cent were in semi-skilled and unskilled work, with a further 36·6 per cent in skilled manual work. This compared with 32 per cent and 38 per cent respectively for the borough as a whole. Some 6 per cent of the population were in the professional/managerial socio-economic group.[1] About half of all the married women in the area were employed, indicating both the scarcity of money in many families and the area's continuing role in servicing the City of London. The Project workers knew of many mothers who had two or three jobs to do in the course of the day, cleaning in the early morning, then perhaps cutting sandwiches for the growing office trade in local shops and pubs, and finally returning to do another cleaning job when the family's evening meal had been prepared. Here we have a widespread example of what we referred to in the first chapter as the internal support resources of families whose male breadwinner is either unemployed or a low-wage earner or whose wages remain relatively fixed against increases in the cost of living.

By age distribution the population was typical of the borough as a whole: 10 per cent of the population was under five years of age, while 11 per cent were 65 or older. The residents were grouped into 10,861 households, a quarter of which were single households (some 2,700 persons lived on their own) of whom well over half were over pensionable age. A notably large section of the population (29 per cent) lived in households of only two persons.

There were other special indicators of need in the Project's target area. One of the best composite measures of need is the number of primary school children who take free meals. The Project found in 1970 that in the two wards (Cathedral and Chaucer) that form the largest part of the Project patch, 18·8 per cent and 24·8 per cent respectively of children of primary school age in the wards took free school meals. Only two wards (one of which, Abbey, is partly located in the Project area) of the twenty-two in the borough had a higher take-up of free school meals. Cathedral, Chaucer and Abbey wards were found, in fact, to have one of the highest concentrations of free school-meal takers and juvenile first offenders. Chaucer and Cathedral wards also had one of the highest rates for stillbirths and infant mortality in the borough.

[1] These figures, and most of those that follow, are taken from the 1966 Census, which was a 10 per cent sample census.

HOUSING

The existing housing stock and housing opportunities comprise one of the most important resources of a neighbourhood. We shall describe the housing stock as the Project found it (i.e. through the Greater London Council Housing Study, 1966), although several buildings were subsequently emptied by collective action taken by tenants. We shall start by giving an overall picture of the housing situation in the Project area and then give some detail about the different types of housing to be found in north-west Southwark.

As a community resource the housing stock was not adequately meeting the demands made upon it. The GLC Housing Study revealed that in Cathedral Ward over a third of dwelling types were tenements, almost 70 per cent of the housing units had been built before 1919, and 35 per cent of dwellings were in 'poor condition'. The figures for the Borough of Southwark were 4·6 per cent, 53·7 per cent and 15·2 per cent respectively. These figures indicate that a large number of households did not possess adequate housing amenities. In the entire Project area, over 5 per cent of households were classified as overcrowded, compared with some 3 per cent in the Borough of Southwark. Indeed, in nineteen census enumeration districts in the area, over 12 per cent of households were overcrowded (i.e. living at more than 1·5 persons per room). Using the GLC index of housing stress, north-west Southwark emerged as one of the areas with the worst housing conditions in the entire borough.

The landlords responsible for the management of most of the housing stock in the area included the local authority, the Greater London Council and the City of London Corporation. Several blocks were owned by housing trusts and some by private companies and individuals. The Church Commissioners and the Church Army were also landlords. The types and quality of housing in the neighbourhood tended to be associated with the kinds of social groups they accommodated. The local authority, the GLC and the Peabody Trust housed, on the whole, relatively stable employed working-class families. The Trust blocks followed the practice of providing housing for the sons and daughters of the present tenants. The tenements, on the other hand, accommodated a heterogeneous population, comprising long-standing residents and recent arrivals in London, some of whom would move into better accommodation but many of whom would stay on living in poverty in single rooms.

The neighbourhood also contained several blocks that were being used as Part III accommodation for homeless families. These included blocks managed by other local authorities such as Lambeth as well as Southwark's Part III accommodation, Chaucer House. Finally, there were hostels in the area that catered for homeless single persons, a group that included both low-wage-earning single men and the dossers and alcoholics who have always been a feature of street life in Southwark. There were also some comparatively recent high blocks of flats in the neighbourhood. Here the tenants were concerned about inadequate play space, poor maintenance, and the loneliness and anxieties of flat-bound mothers with young children.

EMPLOYMENT

Until the 1850s Southwark reaped the benefits of a riverside location and proximity to the City of London. Several markets have prospered in the area, of which the most important is the Borough Market. Hop trading has also been concentrated on and around the riverside and led to the early development of the Courage Brewery and the associated trades of bottling and cooperage.

Docking, wharfage and road haulage have also a long history in north-west Southwark. The wharves have created an elaborate network of ancillary firms in import/export, road transport, ship and barge repair, warehousing, packing and docking.

Printing is another traditional Southwark industry that prospered because of its proximity to the City. The leather, hides and tanning industries are also employers in north-west Southwark, as are the food trades that have been prominent for over a hundred years.

With the growth of the outer suburbs between the two World Wars, firms that no longer required a riverside location and those that required space for expansion and modernisation moved outwards.[1] Between 1961 and 1966, 12,000 industrial jobs disappeared in the London Borough of Southwark. About 5,000 of these jobs disappeared from the northern part of the borough and all the traditional industries were affected. Many more firms moved out

[1] This outline is based on a paper by Dr R. Colenut prepared for the North Southwark Community Development Group.

of north-west Southwark between 1968 and 1972, causing many redundancies because they were relatively large employers and moved far outside the local community.

There was a growing awareness in north-west Southwark of industrial and employment problems as the number of unemployed increased. The most dramatic local issue was the closure of Hays Wharf which lies between London Bridge and Tower Bridge. Between May 1969 and May 1970, Hays laid off 880 workers from their wharves and warehouses in north-west Southwark, and published a scheme for the redevelopment of their land for offices and hotels.

The overall trend has been a decline in employment opportunities in traditional industries and an increase in the number of jobs available in offices. But there was little fit between these kinds of employment opportunities and the skills of north-west Southwark men who, we have already noted, were predominantly blue-collar workers.

THE SERVICE AGENCIES AS RESOURCES

The London Borough of Southwark compared favourably with other Inner London boroughs in terms of its expenditure on most public and social services. It ranked fourth out of twelve Inner London boroughs in 1971-2 for its expenditure per 1,000 population on social services. In the housing field, the return of houses under construction by London boroughs on 31 March 1971 showed that Southwark was building almost two new houses for every one by the London borough with the next highest total.

In this section, we examine some of the services as they operated in north-west Southwark. The Project staff believed that it was necessary to understand this organisational environment and to discover how it was perceived by people living and working in the area and the extent to which the community participated in the planning and design of these services. The Project's primary interest was to assess the needs of the area, to see how services were meeting them and in what ways they could meet them more adequately.

Our analysis of services is organised around five of the basic problem areas that confronted service workers and users. These were:

1 *The Complexity of Services*

The social services in Southwark in 1968 formed a complex web that was poorly understood by the population of the area and by those operating the services. This web consisted of services operated by two tiers of local government, a wide range of voluntary organisations, and central government departments responsible for the health service, probation, the police, pensions, and supplementary insurance benefits.

In 1968, social services for individuals and families in northwest Southwark derived from four departments of the London Borough of Southwark (the Departments of Welfare, Health, Children and Housing); from the Greater London Council Housing Department; and from the Inner London Education Authority (ILEA). These departments had various field work services, residential establishments, day care facilities and other services of various types. In addition, the services provided by voluntary organisations in Southwark were as complex and varied as those in the statutory sphere. Within single departments or organisations particular sections might operate very independently; for instance, this was the case within ILEA with its responsibilities for schools, adult education, youth service, care committees and school enquiry officers.

The difficulties of understanding the complex web of services were compounded by the fact that different agencies had different boundaries, and within agencies (for example, ILEA) there were sections whose boundaries did not coincide.

As far as the public was concerned, it was difficult to obtain information about services and the details of their administration. For example, at the headquarters of most agencies there was no board indicating what was available within the building. From the Project's study of residents' views it appeared that the majority were unaware of most of the existing social welfare facilities. Some exceptions included housing, the police, the doctors, and the Department of Health and Social Security about which general knowledge was more widespread.

Interviews with residents and staff in the information services revealed that people did not know their councillors. Councillors were often confused with employees of council departments. There was little understanding of the structure of local government. The councillors, however, saw themselves as a communication channel for the people.

2 *Variations in the Standards of, and the Need for, Services in Different Localities*

Standards in services varied widely. These variations and differences in the support and servicing of communities became evident from the Project's studies. Variations were attributable to:

a. The different structure and degrees of homogeneity of neighbourhoods. Communities vary in the extent to which they are able to take care of their members' physical, social and psychological needs by mutual support or reserves of resources for crises ('internal support resources'). For example, in neighbouring Bermondsey Project workers were aware of the kinship supports and neighbourly help that played an important part in the local life and which had been labelled 'the Bermondsey spirit'. There was also a close relationship in Bermondsey between local councillors and the local population. But in north-west Southwark the relationship between elected members, the local authority staff, and residents did not appear as significant as the relationship that existed in old Bermondsey.

b. The different ways in which services utilised their resources and applied policies. Public services divide and use their resources and plan their operations to meet crises and to rescue social casualties; or, alternatively, to maintain, protect and support the cohesion of families and to develop the supporting functions of communities. The continuum extends from those services that rescue and contain (e.g. ambulance, long-term residential homes) to the services that promote preventive checks, domiciliary support, community care and neighbourhood involvement. The allocation of resources along this continuum varied from one locality to another and was concentrated on the crises part of the continuum in the Project area.

c. The approach of individuals to their jobs. Where there was fast turnover of field staff, knowledge within departments of local resources was more limited than where the staff had long experience within one locality. Responsiveness to people's situations and demands varied with an individual worker's knowledge of locally available resources and with their approaches to their tasks. It was apparent that workers who were focused on a particular patch and had length of service in the area often knew more about the needs and resources of their locality. There were individual differences between service personnel in their knowledge, skills and attitudes that appeared to determine their ability to be relevant to local needs. The neighbourhood value of individual field workers in services also depended on a number of other factors. Some of these related to their agency: how it was organised; how work was allocated; the extent to which a worker could mobilise required resources; and the extent of the crisis work arising in the locality.

3 Service Capacity to Identify Needs

Many services were not able to meet the needs of all people who were referred to them for help. In addition, there was the 'hidden' need of those who did not or could not apply. Many agencies had clearly defined ideas about which area in their patch they looked upon as being the most needy. They defined need in a variety of ways; for example, from where they got most work, or where they confronted most difficulties in carrying out their particular tasks. Most of these views were related to the staff's personal experience rather than to statistical evidence.

One necessary ingredient in an assessment of the neighbourhood value of services is knowledge of the extent to which they were geared to the most deprived groups. Within the Project area these included:

those living on or below the poverty line;
homeless families and individuals;
transient drug takers, alcoholics, ex-prisoners and mental hospital patients;
physically, mentally and emotionally handicapped people;
those in the worst slum buildings and worst physical environments;
those who needed but did not seek established services or could not use them because of fears or prejudices.

Often, the SCP team were able to identify people who did not make use of the social services but could be classified in one or more of these categories. A coherent social policy did not exist for many of these groups, and for some there were no social services.

The Project found that it was difficult for those in public service in Southwark to focus attention on these groups or on some of the fundamental issues that perpetuated deprivation. Sections within the social services were competing for public support and attempted to do a public relations job to enhance the prestige of their department and, thus, increase their unit's chances of additional resources. This often diverted departments from tackling more basic problems. It seemed easier for officers to attract resources for children's homes, old people's services, holidays for some of the young elderly, and Christmas parcels for the needy, than to tackle more chronic difficulties like those of the 'feckless' or 'anti-social' families and individuals.

4 Planning and Co-ordination Between Services

A major deficiency in service provision was the absence of effective joint structures for planning to meet social deprivation. Other services were usually known to staff on an ad hoc, informal basis. But no machinery existed for joint consideration between departments of issues of common concern such as services to families, services to the old, and services to new communities.

In 1968, most agencies were working in a comparatively isolated manner without regard to related services. This also applied to workers within these services. It was difficult, therefore, for agencies to plan ahead in relation to policy changes that affected their service. For example, when the welfare department closed Newington Lodge, no extra housing units for large families had been agreed with the housing department. This led to more children coming into care within the homeless group.

Inter-organisational work is based on an assumption that there is a need for joint-planning between services to meet human needs and problems more appropriately. The success of those workers in the social services who found some inter-organisational contact to be necessary depended on the proper functioning of the contact networks they had individually developed with others rather than on recognition that this should be a formally structured function.

Some people in organisations at top- or middle-management level considered part of their work to be that of maintaining liaison with other agencies. This was usually done on a case-by-case basis where they wanted to make a referral or bargain for a resource that was available only from some other agency. The traditional 'case conferences' were expensive in labour and often insufficient in effect. They were attempts by agencies and department representatives to sort out a policy for dealing with a family that needed more appropriate help than was readily forthcoming through normal day-to-day mechanisms.

Joint planning between 'helping' services in north-west Southwark required liaison between two tiers of local government, central government, the voluntary services, and neighbourhood interests. Few mechanisms served this purpose in Southwark in 1968. The co-ordinating machinery of officers and members had been set up after the reorganisation of local government services in London in 1965. There was the hope at that time that after reorganisation services would be brought together in a more responsive structure. But shared funding of different services by the same rate-payers under the same council in no way assured the more rational planning of joint programmes.

The same divisions and incoherence found between local authority departments was discovered to exist between the statutory services and the voluntary agencies, who were often dependent on the local authority for funding. Generally, the voluntary agencies felt that the statutory services neglected and ignored their efforts.

5 Change and Reorganisation Within Services

Project workers became aware of a variety of changes affecting local and borough service provision. Changes that occurred during the life of the Project included: central government legislation affecting local services; departmental changes; changes in the political power of groups and individuals in the borough; and staff turnover within the services. These changes were not conducive to forward planning and co-ordination within and between agencies.

New legislation and government budgetary and economic policy, at a time of inflation in food prices and living expenses, affected most severely those in the Project area with low incomes. Examples of this are reductions in benefits and subsidies affecting school children's concessions; the withdrawal of school milk; the trebling in price of school meals; and the reduction of bus fare concessions for journeys to school. There were also increases in prescription and other charges for National Health services and welfare benefits. At the same time, some benefits were added such as the concessionary fares for the elderly and the attendance allowance for the handicapped. The Housing Finance Act had the effect of increasing council house rents for many tenants, and the increase in land and house values in London helped to widen the gulf between the owner-occupier's wealth in Southwark and that of the council tenant or private tenant in the Project area.

Changes in legislation which were meant to influence the local authority's personal social services included the Children and Young Persons Act 1969, and the Chronically Sick and Disabled Persons Act 1970. But the most important in terms of organisational change was the Local Authority Social Services Act 1970. The implementation of this Act involved the integration of most local government social care services into a unified social services department. The Act revealed much need hitherto unmet, at a time when the Chronically Sick and Disabled and the Children and Young Persons Acts led to additional demands on services.

The trauma and upheaval created by such large organisational change began in the latter half of the Project's life. Despite the magnitude of the changes, there was little consultation with staff; agencies were preoccupied with internal problems such as low morale, staff losses and an increasing number of field staff vacancies. These problems, which are features of service provision in many inner city areas, were exacerbated by the reorganisation of the services. During this time, only a few pieces of collaborative work were negotiated by the Project staff with the new department.

There were, too, changes in the local government power structure including turnover in the officers and councillors who had been helpful to SCP in its work with local authority services. In the 'honeymoon' period of the first year, the Project had the patronage of the chief welfare officer, his chairman and some leading councillors with whom the Project's entry to the borough had been negotiated. The town clerk and the children's officer were sympathetic and interested in collaborating with Project staff. Within the first year of Project operations, the chief welfare officer enthusiastically welcomed, and the councillors accepted, the organisation of a Community Development Project in Southwark which was offered by the Home Office. But in May 1969, as a result of local government elections, a number of councillors lost their seats, including some who had supported SCP and who were interested in exploring new community projects. In the same year, the borough lost the town clerk and the chief welfare officer, both of whom had supported the Project. In 1970 the children's officer moved to a post in another borough. The chief officer's power was also altered by the appointment in the middle of 1970 of a chief executive who was new to local government.

THE SCHOOLS AS RESOURCES

Many agencies and services operating in north-west Southwark were attempting to cope with the consequences of the deteriorating housing and employment situations. The primary schools were particularly aware of the difficulties faced by many families who brought their personal problems to the school for help and advice which the head teacher tried to give on an individual basis. There was little contact between the school and the other social service departments except for the school inquiry officers and the voluntary school care committees.

In addition to several state infant schools, junior schools and one girls' secondary school, the north-west area contained a number of church schools founded in the last century with intake from London as a whole. These specialist schools did not relate to the children in the locality and had highly selective intakes. Most local children attended nearby infant and junior schools, although in 1968 children were also allocated to schools further away because of the large numbers of homeless families. For secondary schools, children travelled more widely. A number of infant and junior schools in north-west Southwark had been nominated as EPA schools. Nomination into this category had meant some extra money for staff and equipment. It did not appear to have led to any other major changes in the schools' approaches.

On the whole, staff of schools were working hard to combat the environmental pressures outside and provide a 'sanctuary' for the children who came. The distances travelled by teachers into the area were often long. During the early stages of the Project, teachers staged a one-day strike in which many of them visited the homes of their children for the first time. This had a dramatic effect on some of them and brought home an awareness of the poor housing conditions.

SUMMARY

We can conclude by summarising the major needs and problems of the area as they appeared to the Project and its informants in 1969:

considerable housing need and stress; extreme needs among particular groups of residents such as families in Part III accommodation and single men who slept rough in derelict parts of the area;

continuing decline of local employment opportunities; difficulties for blue-collar workers in adjusting to redundancies and obtaining new work at comparative wage rates;

severe deficiency in open-space provision and inadequate neighbourhood play space;

heavy traffic in the area;

problems of Educational Priority schools struggling with poor facilities and high staff turnover;

problems of loneliness and isolation of mothers with young children resident in two high-rise blocks in the neighbourhood;

planning blight;

decline in the number and variety of shops and other services and the decisions by shops and pubs which remained to cater more to the needs of the day-time working population than to the needs of the residents;

problems and complexities of service provision to an inner city neighbourhood of considerable need at a time services were affected by reorganisation.

The neighbourhood's actual and potential strengths included the work of the Blackfriars Settlement, some local schools, the caring role of the Evelina Children's Hospital and the interaction of the Hospital, Blackfriars workers and the health visitors at the new Health Centre. Two tenants' associations were becoming active in two of the slums and a local member of the Communist Party had begun to enthuse residents in the neighbourhood to take a more direct role in getting the authorities to attend to the needs of the area. One strength for change which was not present was the existence of a home-owning and/or professional group of residents who had the skills and the motivation to 'upgrade' their neighbourhood.

Chapter 3

COMMUNITY ACTORS AND
THE ORGANISATION AND STRUCTURE OF
THE SOUTHWARK COMMUNITY PROJECT

A major theme throughout this book, and a fundamental assumption of much community work practice, is that local communities have much to gain by contributing to the decisions made about community resources. Questions about resource accountability, resource management and participation in decision-making are questions that can also be asked about a community project and, in that vein, we shall describe the internal organisation of the Southwark Community Project.

THE INITIAL PHASE OF INTERVENTION

It became clear in the first year of the SCP that it was potentially as over-committed as many of the other services working in the borough. The SCP had several different commitments. First, it had a commitment to the National Institute to provide teaching and training; it also had commitments to an as-yet-unspecified and unknown local community, to Southwark's social services as well as the expressed desire to co-operate with the local authority on borough-wide issues. The strain of responding to each of these commitments was evident at an early stage. In particular, we find that there was some anxiety amongst Project staff about the allocation of time and energies between the field work and the teaching commitments. There were many team discussions about this issue as workers' preferences and skills became more apparent. On the one hand there was the link with the Institute's teaching programme and the preference of some workers for teaching and research; and on the other hand there was the equally clear need to respond with as many resources as possible to the social problems of a deprived area. The Institute made few teaching demands. These were always agreed upon with the workers and they never took priority over field work needs. It was the workers who wanted to teach and there were differing views among them as to the degree of involvement desirable in the light of the Project's commitment to field work. Project workers also argued that a person's contribution to teaching and study must be related to his own experience in the field. The model, adopted later by the Home Office's Community Development Projects,[1] of separate research and field arms was not followed; analysis and action were seen as inter-related.

The Project was initially accommodated in a settlement as a temporary base for carrying out the ward studies. This was the 'honeymoon' period that the Project experienced with many people and organisations in the borough who struggled to understand what the Project was about and to help the team members in a number of ways. The workers collected a great deal of information and took up the time of a lot of people in an effort to make rational decisions about the work of the Project. During this time the team came to be labelled 'researchers', and it was not easy to make clear that it had not come into the borough with a prescription of what needed to be done.

The team also occupied accommodation in the local authority's welfare department whose chief officer was extremely receptive to the presence of the Project. He asked the team to undertake a study within his department of the policies and procedures for admitting homeless families to Part III accommodation. By the beginning of 1969, the ward studies were nearing completion, and the team moved to the London Bridge area of the borough and allocated work amongst team members. One worker was given the task of working with local service agencies on an inter-organisational and service-development level; her colleague was to concern herself with collaboration with local tenants' groups and to take up borough-wide issues of play and pre-school provisions; the third worker became the link with the neighbouring Blackfriars Settlement and was asked to respond to the chief welfare officer's request for a study of the policies and practices being applied to homeless families.

When the team moved into its neighbourhood shop-front premises a divergence of views about the use of the Project's resources was indicated when some team members began to feel that the Project was focusing insufficiently on work with local residents and groups. This was an extension of prior team discussions

[1] One of which came to Southwark a year after the SCP had started work.

about the desirability of moving into a neighbourhood base which was seen by some team members as the only way in which the SCP could be a resource to residents and in which they could get to know problems of service delivery and liaison. The other view was that an overcommitment to work with neighbourhood groups, who might be in conflict with the local authority, would limit the Project's opportunity to work with that authority's borough-wide services.

TEAM STRUCTURE AND DECISION-MAKING

The structure of the Project had an important effect on the ways in which these kinds of tensions were articulated and decisions were made. The auspices and funding of community work practice are one determinant of its functioning in the field situation. For instance, the reactions of several service agencies to the Project seem to have been influenced by the Project being a part of the National Institute. The chief welfare officer thought that the SCP 'existed to improve training in the social and community work area, whereas the Community Development Project in the middle of the borough was an administrative exercise in effecting co-ordination.' Other people felt that the Project was concerned with research, not only because of the kinds of questions the SCP was asking but also because of its links with the Institute which had just completed a major research project in the borough. It was this research project that also accounted in part for the Health Department's suspicions of the SCP. The presence of workers in service agencies who had trained at the Institute, or who had been refused places on training courses at the Institute, provide two more examples of the way in which the auspices of the Project might have affected the views of service agencies in the borough.

The link-up of the Project with the National Institute had little impact on the relationships between neighbourhood groups and the Project. There was, generally, a low level of concern about what the Institute was and its interests in the promotion of a community work project. Some local residents saw student training and social work as irrelevant to the neighbourhood whilst others welcomed mature students on placement as an additional resource. On rare occasions, people from the area showed interest in the formal constitution of the Institute. The quarterly visits of the Advisory Committee and the Institute letterheads which lay around the office indicated that the Institute provided the auspices for the Project. It was clear to groups that the SCP received no money from the local authority for its work and this helped to establish the credibility of the Project in its alliance with local groups. But, these characteristics of the Institute notwithstanding, residents had little interest.

The Director of the Project was a senior staff member of the National Institute and he reported on the Project's work directly to the Principal of the Institute. One member of the team acted as team leader by virtue of an appointment as senior lecturer at the Institute. As time went by, each team member was perceived by agencies or local groups as 'being in charge' in spite of the fact that the Project attempted to work on a collegiate basis. When issues or conflicts arose, particularly with a service agency in confrontation with a group the Project helped, team members attempted not to respond in a hierarchical fashion. Such issues would not be dealt with by 'the person in charge', nor be referred to the SCP service worker, but would be passed to the community group concerned or to the team member working with that group. Many people in the agencies found this method of work novel, bewildering and frustrating.

Decisions about the work of the Project were taken at weekly team meetings attended by the three workers and the Director and often by students assigned to the Project. At these meetings the staff discussed management problems and made decisions about Project resources and staff work. Team members met quarterly with the Advisory Committee which began to meet in January 1970. This committee was made up of representatives of the Board of Governors and staff members of the National Institute. There was no local authority or neighbourhood representation on the committee. The committee's terms of reference were wide. They included a regular review of the work of the Project and the consideration with Project staff of any issues referred to the committee by either the staff or committee members themselves. The committee was also seen as a channel of communication between the Project staff and the Board of Governors, and the means of representing the responsibilities and interests of the Institute in relation to the Project. The need for this committee resulted from the ever-increasing commitment of the Project to issues in the neighbourhood that brought the Project, because of its work with local groups, into situations of conflict with the local authority.

Project workers felt in these circumstances that the Board of Governors ought to be fully informed of the work of the team more regularly than a yearly report to them by the Project staff would allow.

The committee had an important support role. It also acted on a few occasions as a mediator with the local authority; a meeting with the borough's chief executive particularly facilitated the Project's continued work with service agencies.

TEAM MEETINGS

Team meetings were not designed to steer neighbourhood groups but rather to encourage a team approach, to develop policy and to provide one strand of accountability for field staff. Decisions at these meetings were not about what groups should do, but were largely attempts to inform the workers' activities. Decisions were largely about workers' time and initiatives, decisions the worker would have to make in the course of his practice. The team meeting was an attempt to make these decisions more collective – and hopefully better. It was also used for staff support.

Team meetings were imperfectly recorded so that there is no written account of the changing role and function of the team throughout the life of the Project. It is clear, however, that the team and its individual members did not have any formal control over decisions made by neighbourhood groups that might affect the overall work of the Project. For instance, decisions by local groups to use more aggressive tactics in negotiations with local authority departments often affected the work of Project staff with service agencies. But any loss of this kind in the work with service agencies was accepted where neighbourhood groups were able to strengthen their negotiating position.

A central problem for the team meeting was that it operated outside the ambit of groups and residents whilst individual workers did not. This meant that the team meetings often became a reference group of low priority for the workers. The team meeting operated at one remove from neighbourhood action, and this may have had the consequence of undermining the role of senior workers. The notion of a team leader may not be viable in a situation where workers feel they are accountable to others, notably the community groups. A team leader may feel threatened or confused by his colleagues' accountability to groups, especially if these groups do not participate in decision-making about a project's resources.

Individual workers at the SCP gave different functions and values to team meetings and to the attempt to work on a collegiate basis. Workers responded differently as their various accounts were submitted for analysis and criticism within the team, and as the allocation of time and resources in respect of individuals or the Project was debated. Some workers found this process to be valuable whereas others found it disabling and sought alternative consultation about their work. Some workers felt extremely vulnerable at team meetings. The level of discomfort and vulnerability varied with many factors including the workers' skills and experiences. Those who had previously enjoyed leadership designations in bureaucratic structures found it most difficult to adapt to the rigours of collective decision-making. Likewise, those workers who had relatively little community work experience were the most diffident in sharing knowledge of their work with team members.

There may be something about community work in deprived areas that demands, in a team situation, compatibility of values, ideology, drive and commitment. Within the matrix of anxieties of working within a neighbourhood, and the pressures of a project's work, staff members may become impatient and intolerant of their colleagues who do not care as much, or work as hard or subscribe as passionately, if at all, to certain ideologies about community work and the causes of social and economic deprivation. Some of the workers in the SCP, for instance, were perceived to be less committed to the neighbourhood and its issues and more concerned to document the role behaviour of the community worker as a contribution to the teaching of community work practice. They were also more committed to, and skilled in, the Project's responsibility to train and teach, and to develop thinking in the community work field. These kinds of activities may be sceptically regarded in a community work team which has a strong work ethic and whose limited resources are overburdened in meeting some of the needs of a neighbourhood. When the time and energy of a project's workers are stretched to breaking point, those workers who limit and control their field involvements in order to further a project's training and teaching goals may become the focus of resentment and contempt.

These feelings may be aggravated by other factors: the pace of academic curiosity and subsequent documentation is slower than that of work with neighbourhood groups and service agencies, and this difference may result in friction between team members. It may be that the difference in pace, with accompanying differences in values and commitments, may be accommodated only when a project strictly controls its intake of work to enable team members to develop their interests and skill at their appropriate pace. The absence in a community work project of a policy on work objectives and resources reduces the establishment of work priorities to negotiation and bargaining amongst team members. The struts of various negotiating stances in this situation will depend on factors like the strengths and weaknesses of individual personalities, the sanction of previous work experiences and reputation, and a general sanctimoniousness that seems to attach itself to work with deprived groups.

The history of staff tensions at the Southwark Community Project is in part a history of the team's inability to appreciate the stress to which members were exposed. It is likely that the team underestimated the anxiety and strain endured by workers practising a method of social work intervention that in the late 1960s was relatively untried and unproved in Britain. This was exacerbated by the diverse background of staff members and the fact that casework and academic research in relation to communities was criticised both from within and outside social work. The ongoing criticisms of service agencies in Southwark, which was inherent and explicit in the work of the Project, may have provoked anxieties in those in the Project who had previously worked in similar agencies elsewhere.

There was, too, anxiety for new workers coming into the Project and having to cope with the real or imagined expectations set for them by the previous record of work of the Project, and by the outgoing worker in particular.

The varied styles of work among the members of the SCP team was also a source of anxiety and confusion. Several workers operated in a fairly day-to-day, *ad hoc* manner. Other workers, more accustomed to working in a relatively structured situation such as an agency with more or less clearly defined goals, struggled to achieve and articulate an overall rationale for the Project's existence and its work.

Finally, we must note confusion engendered by the existence of several accountability systems. The Project and its workers were accountable to those in the team with whom they were working, to the National Institute, to service agencies with whom they were collaborating, to neighbourhood groups using the Project, and to their own internal standards of professional behaviour. These different accountability systems produced internal confusion for workers, and aggravated conflict between members in so far as they disagreed over the relative importance of each of these systems.

The team approach has, of course, much to offer community work. The team situation seems to have more potential, if only as a model, for influencing change and growth in the practice of service agencies. The team situation, where it works well, ensures a variety of ideas and creative debate, and provides different perspectives for making decisions affecting a community work project. Inasmuch as decision-making is based on limited information and subjective judgements, the team approach provides checks and balances. The team is also a potential support base for workers because responsibility for decisions is shared and anxieties and dilemmas about work are discussed.

LOCAL PARTICIPATION IN
THE MANAGEMENT OF THE PROJECT

The Project did not establish appropriate structures through which the views of community representatives and the representatives of relevant agencies could be taken into account in the development of the Project's field work. The absence of such structures seems to contrast with the efforts of Project staff to encourage community influence in decision-making about other neighbourhood resources.

There was never any resistance in principle to local participation. But there were a number of factors that the SCP team discussed that led them away from establishing a management structure with local representation. These included:

the difficulty of establishing adequate criteria for choosing representatives, particularly in the early days of the Project when the wrong choice of a local resident or service agency officer would have harmed the development of Project work;
the concern that a management committee composed of residents and agency personnel might divert the committee from its

management function if it became another arena in which to clash on neighbourhood issues;

the concern that service agency representation and the presence of local councillors on a management committee might serve to give disruptive powers to interests with whom neighbourhood groups were in conflict;

the belief that local resident representation in the management of a community work project can confine the project's activities and act against the interest of particular groups in the area. The SCP had to cope, for instance, with the punitive attitudes of some users to the presence of a tenants' association of a homeless family block that received considerable support from the Project;

the fact that local groups were working hard to achieve their own objectives, and it might have been diversionary for groups to concern themselves with problems and issues other than their own;

the apprehension that a management structure that co-existed with team meetings would have no effective decision-making responsibilities. We have already noted that the nature of much of the SCP's work placed decision-making in the hands of individual workers and the team meetings.

The failure to provide a management structure in which local people could have participated may have made it harder for local groups to accept responsibility and management for the Project when its original auspices and funds terminated.

Another consequence of the organisational structure of the SCP was that the field workers were forced to treat neighbourhood groups in ways they would have avoided in other contexts. In discussions, for instance, about the existing work load of the Project and whether or not new invitations to work ought to be taken up, it was often necessary to make some assessment of the existing and anticipated needs of local groups and residents. Because no local residents were present, workers acted in effect as spokesmen for the groups, a role that workers did tend not to take when groups were dealing with third parties like one of the local authority services. There were many occasions in the life of the Project when local people, usually officers of groups using SCP services, sought some kind of control or influence over SCP decision-making, and there were times when local people disagreed with decisions made by staff. Residents had few sanctions to impose on the Project on the occasion when disagreements arose over Project policies and decisions. Groups could, of course, stop using the Project, though this was not a real sanction because the kinds of services available in the Project were not readily available from other organisations in the neighbourhood. Thus, there was no reality to the notion of consumer choice even in regard to use of the Project, though later, in the 1970s, more community workers were available in the area. There were, on the other hand, some instances in the course of the SCP when officers of groups stayed away from the Project to show their displeasure with Project decisions.

The absence of a management body with local representation involved the workers in the Project in some ambiguous situations. For example, neighbourhood groups sometimes sought to influence the direction of Project business by passing on their views and grievances to the staff member in the Project with whom they worked. Whether or not this was an effective way of influencing a discussion depended in part on whether the worker subscribed to the views of the groups which were themselves seldom unanimous. The confidence that developed between workers and groups made it possible for this procedure to work sometimes. However, when a worker left the Project, groups lost this channel of influence within the Project. Thus, at such times, when the impact of a new worker portended changes, Project users lacked an influential voice in decision-making.

In a later chapter we shall look at the services offered to the community by the Project and consider how relevant they continued to be to the needs of groups and families living in the community. In this section an attempt has been made to highlight some of the effects of administrating a neighbourhood resource in such a way that it divorces the community development opportunities presented in its own organisation from the services it provides in the field which are concerned precisely with opening up those self-same opportunities in the action groups to which people belong.

Local groups, through their negotiations with the local authority and through their contact with the Project, acquired skills by which to scrutinise resources and the agencies responsible for the administration of those resources. Several groups developed a critical awareness of the services and limitations of resources working in, or on behalf of, their neighbourhood. The Project was able both to assist in promoting this sense of scrutiny and to resist (because of the workers' judgement in the matter) any change in the Project itself that users may have wanted to suggest as a result of their keener appreciation of the relationship between a resource and neighbourhood needs and values.

THE DUAL APPROACH: WORKING WITH SERVICES AND WITH NEIGHBOURHOOD GROUPS

The broad choices open to the SCP team about the allocation of their time and resources were:

to work primarily with neighbourhood groups and through them to effect changes in agency services;
to work primarily with service agencies at a number of different levels; or
to work with community groups but at the same time attempt to work directly with services.

The Project chose the third option, which the team referred to as 'the dual approach'. A detailed analysis of work with service agencies comes in Chapter 8; in this section we discuss some of the problems and strains of a dual approach.

An important question confronting a community work agency that adopts the dual approach is: Will the agency's work with neighbourhood groups affect its collaboration with services, and vice versa? As far as residents using the SCP were concerned, work undertaken with services did not appear to be dysfunctional to neighbourhood work. Residents were often curious about what workers were doing with service people and asked about those who visited the Project. Sometimes this led to new contacts being made between the agency staff and the residents. One of the major reasons why neighbourhood work did not suffer was because the team gave priority to the residents and neighbourhood affairs. In the interests of residents' achievements the team often refrained from pushing forward their work with services. For example, little work was done to bring the services together in the immediate locality of the Project where most groups using the Project were located. On the other side, the Project's collaboration with groups like the squatters and tenants' associations concerned with slum clearance constrained the efforts of the SCP service worker.

Tenants' associations sometimes used information collected by the Project in work with services. This had interesting repercussions. For example, a report on homeless families was seen in the flat of the chairman of a tenants' association in a Part III block by a health visitor who was shocked that this information was available to the tenants' association. The worker attempted to explain to the health visitor that the tenants' association was as important as others who were concerned about the effects of homelessness and had been one of the providers of information. It also had the opportunity to take action that was not always open to agency staff.

The dual approach seemed to facilitate interaction between community groups and service agencies. For example, many community groups affected agencies' behaviour and policies by negotiations with chief officers and councillors. In other instances, agency staff and community representatives joined together to consider issues and pursue action, for instance, in relation to services for the young handicapped, and to improve the prevention of homelessness.

The potential power of the community voice as a political tool for agency interests was also apparent. At various stages in the Rockingham Estate Multi-Service Group, the tenants' association was asked to intervene or take action in ways they did not find desirable, as the following illustrates:

'The Chief Executive's Project Team has apparently had continuing difficulties with the Greater London Council in agreeing on the use of the land which they jointly own, on which the Multi-Service Centre could be built. The tenants' association have been asked to prevent them building the community hall part separately. Apparently the other services feel that the pressure of the tenants' association could tip the balance. It is interesting that the association has refused to be used as a tool. They have fought for three years for a community hall and to write now saying stop building to the GLC was considered not to be in the interest of the residents.'

Once they were organised, many neighbourhood groups received requests for help from various services: for example, Mint Street Playground Committee gave permission to a local headmaster to use their football pitch; the Rockingham Estate Community was asked for help by several agencies in relation to 'at risk' elderly individuals. But some service requests were considered by local groups to be inappropriate, such as when they were asked by agency staff to undertake menial jobs (e.g. laying lino, cleaning neglected flats). Such requests confirmed some residents' fears that the service providers undervalued and misunderstood the role they should play.

The benefits of the dual approach were maximised where close communication and common values existed among SCP team members; when information was regularly shared the possibility of conflicting actions could be minimised. Each person had to make special efforts to keep abreast of developments in the work of others and share information about important changes they encountered so that confusions and tensions would not occur.

In some situations it was possible for the same team member to work with services and community groups on the one issue simultaneously. This was particularly true if conflict was not too great. But in the field of slum housing clearance and homelessness, separation of functions between SCP workers was seen as more likely to achieve changes because conflict was so intense. The dual approach also allowed agency staff and people from the neighbourhood to divide the Project workers into 'goodies and baddies'. Agency staff often tried to use the Project service worker to control the neighbourhood workers. There were, too, occasions when service personnel sought to use a Project worker as an intermediary to resolve a dispute with a community group.

The continuing interplay between work with services and neighbourhood groups is reported throughout the remainder of this book. The picture emerges of the Project service worker attempting by a variety of interventions to influence services within the constraints for change set by the SCP's work with local residents and by the insularity of the social services in a period of reorganisation. The local residents, however, provided a constituency for the Project's work with services even though many residents did not understand, or were suspicious of, contacts with agencies. The Project service worker waged a less dramatic and visible campaign than those who worked with community groups. This was a campaign of attrition consisting of persistence in helping staff of services to relate their resources rationally to the area, to study and to plan within and between departments, to identify with neighbourhood problems and to see the community's inhabitants as whole persons rather than as cases for a particular form of social

service provision. It would be a major achievement of this work
with services if the voluntary and statutory agencies in the borough
have become more ready to understand and to incorporate consumers' own views of their needs and of service provision. This
leaves in question the role of the elected representative.

WORK WITH ELECTED REPRESENTATIVES

Systematic work with councillors was not a feature of the Project's
intervention in north-west Southwark. This is accounted for partly
by a number of conscious decisions by the Project that were based
on the possible effects that working with councillors might have
had on relationships with officers and neighbourhood groups; and
partly by the fact that councillors in north-west Southwark did not
appear to be a significant factor in the political and community
lives of the neighbourhood's residents. Southwark as a whole is
an overwhelmingly Labour-controlled constituency, and an important aspect of borough political life is the poor participation of
the electorate in local and general elections. Together with
boroughs like Tower Hamlets and Hackney, Southwark has one of
the lowest election turn-outs of all London boroughs. Within
Southwark itself, the average for the borough of those voting in
local elections was 31·1 per cent whereas the percentage voting
in Cathedral ward was as low as 19·0 per cent (May 1971).

The Southwark Community Project and its user groups interacted with members and officers both of the local authority in
Southwark and of the Greater London Council, but more especially
with the former. Project workers found in Southwark that the
role of a councillor was likely to be determined by a variety of
factors including:

the individual preferences and abilities of councillors;
the view held by many councillors and officers that local government is concerned with the narrow provision of a series of services rather than with the overall well-being of local communities;
the nature and extent of problems in councillors' own constituencies. It appeared that many councillors were driven by a
sense of hopelessness away from the seeming intractability of
'local problems' towards borough-wide or town hall issues;

the satisfaction gained by councillors from work with individual
constituents;
the tendency to view local responsibility primarily in terms of
the interests of individual constituents;
the lack of any political or administrative machinery at the local
level.

The role of many councillors in north-west Southwark as local
representatives was largely concerned with the problems of individual families as they were presented by letter or on the street,
or in promoting or participating in public meetings to explain a
specific council proposal for the neighbourhood. Most of these
councillors saw their wards as 'isolated and apathetic'. One councillor remarked that 'the community do not use me much'. He had
relatively few letters from constituents, and he complained of the
widespread apathy and poor turn-out at elections; most of the ward,
he suspected, did not know of his existence. Most community action in the area seemed to pass the councillors by, though there
were often occasions when a tenants' group would use a councillor
to chase up a chief officer or to pursue the housing problem of an
individual tenant. Several of the councillors who were helpful to
the Project and to local groups were from wards in the southern
part of the borough.

Monthly meetings of the ward Labour Party in Cathedral were
poorly attended. There was no local councillors' surgery and constituents had to trek to the Walworth Road in order to find a
surgery that served the needs of the whole borough . . . and that
one on Friday evenings only. Several councillors felt that they
knew the people and their problems but there was little evidence
that this feeling was reciprocal. A survey on one estate in 1969
interviewed eighty-eight tenants, of whom only three said they
knew a local councillor. Two of these three were not able to name
the councillors they knew. In a question about problems and complaints, no tenant mentioned going for advice to a councillor.

Along with the low turn-out at elections in the area, these findings seem to indicate that many residents did not see councillors
as relevant community resources. It also seems to be the case that
councillors may have underestimated the resources of their own
constituents. The presence of councillors with inappropriate or
ineffective roles in a constituency that has become indifferent to
political process may allow for the perpetuation of neighbourhood

problems and may undermine the accountability of elected members and officers to local communities. It also exposes that local authority in its policy-making to the influences of parties in the authority's area who have identified their self-interest and are able to pursue it articulately such as constituencies of owner-occupiers, and high-rate yielding businesses. We found in 1972, for instance, that Southwark was having regular discussions with property companies in order to work out redevelopment plans for north-west Southwark with little attempt on the part of officers or councillors to involve local residents and obtain their views on the redevelopment of their neighbourhood.

The Project's contacts with councillors in Southwark began when discussions of the Project's entry to the borough were undertaken with the leader of the council and some of his colleagues. As work with neighbourhood groups developed, it became Project policy for both neighbourhood and service groups to approach councillors about issues that concerned them. Although local councillors appeared relatively unknown to residents, groups regularly used contacts with influential councillors (e.g. with the chairman of appropriate committees) once they discovered how to achieve success. From time to time the SCP team had contacts with councillors at a fairly marginal level. Councillors were invited to meetings and events that were held at the Project, but the team did not otherwise seek to provide them with information and help except through the circulation of surveys and documents about the area.

One reason why the team did not try harder with councillors was that it feared adverse consequences for their work with the community groups. Another concern lay in the Project's involvement with officers of the council and there may have been further constraints on officers' responses had the workers been allied with councillors in any meaningful way.

In discussing whether to work more closely with local councillors, the team had also to consider that much of its neighbourhood work was in relation to slum clearance and the rehousing of residents, mostly outside the area. Such constraints might not have been of major interest to councillors. But where local groups were likely to make some long-standing impact (e.g. the adventure playgrounds), councillors sought to associate themselves with the activity and to acknowledge the group's usefulness.

Most of the councillors representing north-west Southwark had lived there all their lives and had been councillors for many years. They probably felt ambivalent towards the intervention of professional 'outsiders' who sought and achieved politically-orientated alliances with groups of constituents. The conflicts initiated by neighbourhood groups with officers and chairmen of the local authority's departments may also have been threatening to councillors who thought that they knew 'what the people want'. Councillors may have resented not only the success of groups such as tenants' associations and playground committees in effecting neighbourhood changes, but also the fact that the achievement of such changes was emblematic of a gulf between councillors and residents. Many local people began to perceive that their tenants' association was a more pertinent force for change than their elected representatives. Local councillors did not appear to see the power of local groups as a healthy stimulus to their own efforts or as a necessary check on centralised decision-making.

It may be more difficult for a councillor to intervene in the collective lives of his constituents than it is for a stranger like the community worker. In many working-class communities public service is often associated with personal advancement and prestige. It is perhaps much easier for residents to accept the leadership of another resident than the leadership of a councillor. The former appears to serve no other interest than his own which is similar to the collective interest such as to attain better housing. The councillor may be cynically seen as wanting to secure his own advancement. The situation is, of course, never as clear as this. The tenants' chairman may be rehoused more quickly and in a better flat, and he may enjoy having his name in the paper. But these are often seen as perks of the job, justified by considerable self-sacrifice and few of his constituents will resent them or view them cynically. Because local councillors represent a large constituency, and because they are often absent from the ward in order to be at the town hall, residents will not be as aware of the enormous demands made upon a councillor's time and energies.

These competing demands form the crux of the dilemma facing local councillors. They have limited time in which to carry out their duties at the town hall, to deal with individual cases for advice or help, and to become a familiar person in their wards, assisting and encouraging the work of local groups.

Chapter 4

SOME OPENING MOVES IN
NEIGHBOURHOOD WORK

The task of identifying local issues is one of the most difficult encountered by the novice community worker. He is quite insecure and uncertain about his tasks, exploring a new role, and feeling grave doubts about his authorisation for intervening in the life of the community. Experienced workers share some of the same anxieties in the early stages of community work. Immediate answers are required for the following sort of questions: How do you approach people? Do I knock on a door or stop someone in the street?; How will I introduce myself?; Will they understand what I say?; Will they talk to me?; What business have I to confront local people about problems in their area? Whilst it is all right for male community workers to knock on doors and approach strangers, what do they think when they see me, a woman, engaged in these activities?

BECOMING ACQUAINTED

In discussing these issues it is useful to distinguish between the time when a community worker first comes into an area, and the later stages when a worker, already established, makes efforts to contact particular groups, such as residents on an estate, or immigrant adolescents, or vagrants. In the earlier stages, he will be concerned to build a store of knowledge about the neighbourhood. The worker will talk to professionals in the neighbourhood (e.g. priests, teachers, police, probation officers) as well as to those in the local authority who are responsible for that area. There is, of course, relatively little difficulty for the worker in approaching his peers in other professions and services. On the other hand, it is not unlikely that the worker, as he abandons his desk for the street, will feel that although some people may want to talk to him, many are hostile to, or suspicious of, or indifferent to him. He may even be unsure of his own motivations. He might feel, often rightly, that his way, his voice, his clothes and his bearing will mark him off as 'one of them', some part of officialdom to be treated with caution. His self-doubts may be based on a lack of awareness of the function of the street and the pavements as a forum for conversation and interaction between neighbours and friends and between residents and the strangers that pass through the neighbourhood. Jane Jacobs has expressed this very clearly:

'People's love of watching activity and other people is constantly evident in cities everywhere. . . . A lively street always has both its users and pure watchers. Last year I was on such a street in the lower east side of Manhattan waiting for a bus. I had not been there longer than a minute . . . when my attention was attracted by a woman who opened a window on the third floor of a tenement across the street and vigorously yoohooed at me. . . . She shouted down "The bus doesn't run here on Saturdays. . . ." Then by a combination of shouts and pantomime she directed me around the corner. This woman was one of the thousands upon thousands of people who casually take care of the streets. They help strangers. They observe everything that is going on.'[1]

If there is an active street life in a community, the worker can be quite passive, letting people make contact with him, creating opportunities that allow others to express their caring and curiosity. These opportunities may be fashioned in a number of ways, such as waiting at a bus stop and looking uncertain about places and directions. Project workers, for instance, found that by carrying street maps they provided opportunities for residents to initiate contact. For instance, a worker recorded:

'I talked in the street to a man in his fifties, who asked me if I had lost my way. He started talking about the Aylesbury clearance, and he complained bitterly about the dust and dirt. . . . In the Church Commissioner's estate, as I was standing looking at a map, an elderly man came out of his house and asked if I was the man who was going to take his garden away. . . . An old man was standing near . . . he asked me if he could help me with my map.'

[1] Jane Jacobs, pp. 47–8. *The Death and Life of Great American Cities* (Penguin, London 1972).

Carrying a map was a useful means of expressing the worker's need for information and assistance, leaving the initiative to others to open the conversation. Once initiated, the workers were able to develop the encounters in ways that allowed the residents to talk easily. These contacts on a busy street or in the courtyard of a block of flats were expanded to include friends and neighbours passing by, so that the worker's perception of the neighbourhood or the estate was enlarged and diversified. In addition, there were often people on the streets, especially in the summer, who were looking for contacts and conversation. One worker wrote:

'Much of the area is long established and many people stopped me in the road to ask me what I was doing or whether I was about to call on their house when they were going out shopping. Some had been in the area for thirty or forty years and were obviously worried about the possibility of having to move away from it. A number of the older people said that they had seen the area deteriorate somewhat. There was a very great sense of friendliness and a number of people stopped to speak to me and asked if I had lost my way and four people in a row came up to me and asked, in a more aggressive way, what I was doing and who I worked for. One of these was a dustman who worked in the same area for the past ten years, and the three others were housewives. At one point, I also had a rather nice comment from an old age pensioner. As I passed by, she turned to her friend and said, "They do a lot of drawing but they don't make the traffic any better." '

The SCP workers found that it was advisable to avoid accosting individuals and blurting out 'I am from the Project and wondering what people feel about this neighbourhood'. They often found it better to adopt a more passive role, creating opportunities and pretexts for others to initiate contact, waiting for views on the area to develop from a more casual and general conversation. Residents' views are likely to be more honest and real when they find their expression in these ways than in responses given to strangers who ask outright for them. This became apparent very quickly to one student who wrote:

'My next move was to start doing the door to door approach and at the same time selling *Clarion*, a local newspaper produced by community groups in the area. I think that there is an opportunity of using the sale of the paper to build a relationship which allows an easier mode of communication. I mean by this that residents will feel able to talk to someone they know in a non-threatening contact, to talk of problems. . . . I was able to try another survey of the area when circulating leaflets . . . and on practically every street someone was willing to allow me to use the leaflet as the opening to discussion on the wider issues of being a tenant of the estate.'[1]

Of course, there are initiatives that a community worker can take that carry no threat to the residents or demands for knowledge; a worker can ask for the time, or for street directions. Success here is likely to depend on variables like the worker's appearance and bearing, the degree of activity and friendliness in the street, and the weather.

Local contacts can be made in some of the public areas of the community such as cafes, shops, launderettes and public houses. The public house near to the Project's office was often a useful point of contact in the community. Like the cafe and the small shops, the pub gives the investigating worker a relatively unambiguous locus and an opportunity to gain knowledge and meet people in a relaxed and informal social atmosphere. The worker can also use his links with persons like publicans and shopkeepers to meet others. The worker's introduction of himself to additional people may be facilitated if he can claim that 'Mr Jones at the corner shop suggested that I get in touch with you'. For example, a Project worker wrote:

'I talked with Joe, the proprietor of the paper shop. . . . For further information he recommended me to Mr Mathias, the caretaker. I was to mention Joe's name. . . . The Crown was within fifty yards of Arcadia. . . . Mr Ballantine, the proprietor, knows a number of the families. . . . For further information see the Williams family. Old Mr Williams is dead but his widow and two other sons still live there. Mention Mr Ballantine to them.'

Knowledge and opportunities for work at the neighbourhood level were also acquired by linking up with professionals already

[1] This student was not on placement at the Southwark Community Project but in a neighbourhood association in south London.

established in the area whose gatekeeper functions were similar to those of the publican and the shopkeeper.

Introductions to residents and neighbourhood groups in north-west Southwark were also achieved by going to public meetings in the area called by established professionals and other community groups and organisations. At the same time, residents themselves acted in this capacity and the SCP workers were often referred down through a line of friends and neighbours as they attempted to build up knowledge and local contacts. They realised that a professional such as a clergyman who has built up a wide range of contacts in the community can be useful in introducing the new worker to local people.

One of the consequences for the worker of establishing his presence in the neighbourhood is that initiatives for organising work will become available to him. The following passage indicates an example of this:

'Alan, a local curate, has contacted the Project asking for a member to become involved with him in working with homeless families at Chaucer House, as they were forming a residents' association. . . . After meeting Alan, it was decided that I attend a public meeting of the association, and Alan introduced me as Jill from the Community Project. When I arrived at the meeting I was quite prepared to sit in the audience and perhaps make a short speech about the Project, but when Alan introduced me to the secretary and chairman they both insisted that I sit with them in front of the meeting, and I spoke about the Project. . . . At a difficult point in the meeting the chairman asked me to read out the list of grievances although I would have preferred her to do this because I felt it would be wrong for me to take too much initiative; yet perhaps my reading of the list of grievances was a good introduction of myself to the group.'

In brief, the community worker uses the links and the intro-ductions provided by his various contacts with the neighbourhood to explain himself as a resource either to groups or to local residents inclined to collective action on an issue that concerns them. More-over, he will use his relationships with the professional workers in the area to recruit members for particular groups. For example, an SCP team member approached a local curate who was interested in play facilities. She wrote:

'I met him and found that he lived in a flat overlooking the very site which the Planning Department hoped to use for play space. He immediately thought of several people he knew who would be interested in knowing that the site might be proposed as some form of open space and agreed to see whether they felt that any action should be taken. As part of his effort, he approached the Red Cross Way Tenants' Association. At the same time I had also been in touch with the Queens Building Tenants' Association, and in particular with one very able and hard-working member who became active encouraging members of the committee to support the attempts to get better play facilities in the area.'

The local Press is another mechanism through which a worker becomes engaged with groups and unorganised people in the area. The local newspaper may report the complaints of residents about their housing conditions or environment. If these issues seem likely to accord with the priorities of the agency, the worker might use the newspaper report as an invitation to make contact with the residents concerned. Likewise, a worker can scrutinise other information sources for opportunities to intervene on issues that are of interest to him and his agency. For instance, one worker came to the Southwark Community Project with an interest in vandalism and was able to identify from a survey of local Press reports the estates that seemed to have problems with damage to property.

In the following sections of this chapter, we will describe how the community worker begins the process of group formation. It will be useful here to distinguish between two different situations: the first is one in which the worker's goal is to generate group action in respect of a specfic issue; in the second situation, the goal of the worker is to enable a specific group of people to organise for community action. The distinction is, of course, only for the purposes of discussion. In reality the worker may have varying degrees of goal specificity in respect of both the issues for action and the population to be organised. However, the distinction does allow us to consider different aspects of community work practice. In the first situation, where there is population specificity, the worker has a good sense of *whom he wants to organise* (e.g. the tenants of a housing estate) and his tasks are to determine the pragmatic means by which to do so. In the second situation, where there is issue specificity, the worker knows he wants to do something about a *particular problem* (e.g. poor housing, lack of recreational facilties) and his major methodological tasks are the identification and recruitment of appropriate individuals, groups and organisations. We should note, in passing, that these practice concerns were especially prominent in the early stages of the Project. Later on, many individuals and groups came to the Project on their own initiative to request assistance in organising around different issues and/or to achieve greater cohesion within their groups and organisations.

ORGANISING A SPECIFIC POPULATION

This section is largely about community work intervention in blocks of flats and flatted housing estates, because these were the major types of housing in the target area of the Project. The community life of such areas does not afford workers the variety of opportunities for informal public social interaction that exists in the street situation. On estates, we do not find a juxtaposition of housing with services like pubs, shops and cafes. On estates, we do not find the quantity and variety of contacts among tenants in public places that occurs on streets. The balconies or walkways or public squares or yards that are common in most estates do not appear to promote the degree of informal social interaction that takes place in the street between neighbours and, more importantly from our viewpoint, between residents and strangers amongst whom we must count the community worker.

We start by looking at the activities of a Project worker on a large post-war Greater London Council estate. This estate was chosen in order to investigate the needs and opportunities for community work in a setting which appeared to lack the severe pressures of housing stress present in several other settings in which the Project was already working. The worker developed three lines of action in making his contacts on the estate. First, he took a preliminary walk around the estate to get the feel of the place and noted the kinds of accommodation it provided. Second, he examined the available census data for the enumeration districts which included the estate. And third, he studied the Project files and discovered that there was a tenants' association, known as the the estate's 'social club'. Tony, the worker, went to interview the club secretary. Tony explained who he was and what the Project was about, and expressed an interest in learning about life on the estate. The secretary gave him a friendly and considerate reception and also suggested some other people with whom he might talk.

Armed with these suggestions, Tony conducted further informal interviews on the estate. He first contacted the caretakers, from whom he obtained additional names of residents, and the estate-based clergy before making informal contacts with individual residents.

Thus, with a limited investment of time, about six fieldwork days, the worker managed to gain an initial entrée into the estate and had obtained a general picture of its social structure and services problem. The interviews revealed that the estate did indeed have community problems. These included: few facilities for children on the estate; lack of residents' support for estate activities; isolation of old people; and the unreliability of lifts and heating. The social club treasurer had also expressed the need for more information and hoped that Tony would be able to inform him about the opinions of people on the estate, particularly the newcomers. The leader of the under-fives playgroup on the estate gave the worker the names of three mothers of children at the play centre to whom she suggested it might be useful to talk. His visit to these mothers served to broaden his view of the estate. The interviews brought to light that residents had made efforts to improve the estate. They had, for example, petitioned the council to provide play facilities. These interviews were supplemented by informal contacts in the estate launderette with a few pensioners. They highlighted the lack of amenities for pensioners, particularly the need for benches for sitting out.

Selection of Issues

The work had now reached the stage at which the community worker could select one of the issues that had been thrown up and begin to organise for social action. In taking this step, it is important to be clear that the issue selected is not chosen simply because it appeals to the community worker and suits his values. For one thing, it is necessarry to know whether it is an issue that is relevant to more than just a few of the residents whom the worker happened to contact. It may be that some community work will deal with unpopular or minority issues and reflect the individual community worker's own values and interests. However, in selecting issues one must be aware of what other salient issues are being rejected and how widespread the concern with these may be. In selecting an issue to run with, the community worker needs to be concerned with whether it is relevant. The question might be more pointedly stated as: 'relevant for whom?' – for the old person one has met in the laundry or pub, or relevant for the community worker and his values and beliefs, or relevant for a sizeable proportion of residents on the estate? If it is not of concern to sufficient numbers of residents the worker may find it difficult to get support for some sort of initiative or group.

The Project worker decided not to move directly into an action stance to generate support for one of the issues mentioned, but to check out initial impressions and informal data by conducting a survey of a systematic sample of residents. The worker faced five essential decisions:

deciding on the type of survey;
determining the size and nature of the sample;
framing the questions;
alerting the respondents;
tabulating the survey.

The worker decided to use face-to-face interviews with respondents in their homes. A face-to-face survey offered the worker a chance to talk with local people and to see for himself the conditions in which they lived. This type of survey also enabled the worker to size up the respondents and to identify those who might be motivated to join in some collective action. The face-to-face encounter also gave the worker the opportunity to discover what tenants might be able to contribute to collective action, e.g. their leadership potential, articulateness, community experience, and reputation on the estate.

The worker decided on a quota sample of residents which would reflect the composition of the estate. A 10 per cent sample was obtained from a card file held by the parish church of each household on the estate known to the church. Using the card file, the worker selected households of each type sufficient to constitute the quota sample. Lacking the parish card file, the worker could have used other resources in drawing up the quota including census data, the material at the rent office where tenancy agreements show family composition, and the help of local people such as the caretaker and residents. Local people could have been asked to help the worker list the sorts of households in each flat or building. To do this the worker might actually have gone to each of the buildings with the residents so that they could jog their memories. Other local sources would include caretakers, the milkman, play-group leaders, pool collectors, and insurance agents. From these various sources a quota sample could have been produced.

For the conduct of the interviews, a card of twenty issues was prepared to present to the residents from which they were asked to pick the three issues of central concern to them. In making his initial contacts, the worker had witnessed the anxiety of some residents, especially old-age pensioners, about opening their doors to strangers. The local paper covered stories of robberies of unsuspecting people by strangers knocking at their doors. To help allay these fears and to increase the likelihood of obtaining co-operation from the sample, the Project worker decided to send to each household some advance notification of his intended visit. He spent some time composing a message. To increase the possibility of a message being read, and hopefully retained in the house as a reminder, he limited the message to a postcard. Accepting this limit, he decided he would have to say who he was (and who he was not, e.g. that he was not from the council), indicate what he was about and what he wanted from the residents. In composing the message he tried to avoid using words or phrases that might denote an official status or activity such as 'your co-operation is requested', or 'we are conducting a small survey'. In short, he sought to be both clear and non-threatening. To add a personal touch and further dispel any possibility of an official aura to the cards, he addressed them by hand.

The Intervention Phase

When the survey was completed and the results tabulated, the Project worker considered the question of how he should proceed from the information-gathering phase to intervention. He was not committed to focus on any predetermined problems. He had not been asked by any outside body or authority to enter the estate with particular terms of reference. Similarly, he had not been invited to work on the estate by the residents, although the secretary of the social club had indicated his concern with the problems of non-participation. Neither had the worker attempted to involve residents in carrying out the survey because he did not know beforehand that there would be issues of sufficient interest to warrant a community work initiative. He had entered the estate with the question of the possibility and nature of his involvement left open until the survey was completed. However, after the survey he was certain that there were issues facing residents on which action could be taken.

While community workers may believe that the selection of issues should properly be left to participants, the Project worker encountered practical difficulties in implementing this belief. As with any large assembly of individuals, residents of the estate did not speak with a single voice about the issues of concern to them. The social committee, for example, was concerned with providing social activities for an essentially middle-age group. In contrast, some of the newer residents on the estate, generally younger families, were concerned with quite different matters.

The worker's next move was to feed back his findings to the community. He began by discussing the survey findings with the two clergymen who had let him use their card file to compile the quota sample. Following this meeting, the worker revisited one of the residents, who had a particular knowledge of the estate, to discuss the findings with her. A short list of potential participants for some form of future action programme was drawn up from those who had been interviewed in the survey. Those who were most interested and seemed most experienced or articulate were selected. The worker then revisited these people to discuss the findings, to test the degree of their interest in a programme and to enlist their support for some sort of meeting. The worker also wrote to everyone who had been interviewed with a summary of the survey findings. This decision reflected the growing practice of offering recognition and thanks to those who give their time and opinions to researchers. In addition, it was thought that this was another means of heightening interest on the estate in the issues that had been raised, another means by which the worker could help to create a 'community of concern' among the often disparate residents, each walled off in their own flat perhaps unaware that others on the estate shared their concerns.

The third planning decision was to press ahead with efforts to contact other local people who might assist in whatever work might emerge. Potential leverage points within the social committee were to be followed up and some of the people first contacted who had expressed interest in the survey were to be revisited in order to try to bring together a small group of highly motivated residents, since the worker thought that the chances of success in organising and deciding on next steps would be greater than if he worked with a large assembly of individuals brought together in a public meeting. The results of the revisits were agreements from members of five households to attend a small meeting, and the worker's next move was to pick a night that seemed suitable for most people, as well as a place in which to hold the meeting.

This brief summary[1] of the initial steps in an intervention on a post-war estate has been presented in some detail because it contains some interesting and fruitful description of the kinds of decisions community workers are called upon to make when attempting to gain entry into a community. It might be helpful to present some of the thoughts and decisions that guided the worker in the situations he confronted on this post-war estate. For instance, the worker had to make some advance plans for the first small meeting of residents, and similar planning had to be done for any action that was taken afterwards. Conflict and consensus were the twin strategies that presented themselves to him. However, he also recognised that the choice of strategy was not really his to make. Questions about the role of the worker in determining strategy often face workers when operating with a residents' group. For example, a residents' group is to meet but the specific outcome is uncertain. As a community worker, one may be tempted to espouse a particular course and enter the meeting with one's own agenda, seeking in the meeting to bring off the outcome that one has decided upon. Alternatively, a worker could see the uncertainty of outcome as a positive feature, with the residents entering a situation where they have the power to decide the outcome in terms that make sense to them. This latter view requires that the worker abandon attempts to control the situation, that he leaves his agenda at home.

In practice, the alternatives may be seldom so clear, but it may help the community worker if he himself is clear about this matter and he shares his approach with the group; for example, he might put forward a particular course of action but indicate that this is only one possible course.

Some community workers may offer no opinion even when called upon. Although this offers the comfort of keeping one's hands clean

---

[1] Taken from a paper prepared for the Southwark Community Project by Harley D. Frank, *Facilitating Social Change on an Urban Housing Estate.*

from charges of manipulation, the group might interpret the worker's behaviour as not caring about them or their problem, or as hostile; the group may interpret the worker's behaviour as a refusal to help the committee with its tasks. Another possibility is for the worker to steer away from taking sides on an issue, acting as a clarifier of others' contributions, amplifying them, and translating them into other terms if they are misunderstood. Further, he might spell out some of the consequences of the various points put forward, leaving the meeting to decide what action should be taken.

The absence of indigenous involvement in carrying out the survey should be noted. Project records indicate that the worker considered the survey to be an information-gathering instrument and not a community work intervention. An important question to consider is how the activity of information-gathering creates expectations in the target group and a sense of engagement in the mind of the worker. From this point of view it may not be appropriate to regard information-gathering as distinct from other community work activity. Indigenous involvement in the survey might be a way to gain the co-operation and confidence of tenants and to generate sustained discussion on some of the issues. If tenants co-operate with the worker at this stage of his intervention, helping him with the survey, they will be more connected to any future action and better able to control and discuss the findings of the survey. If the survey is seen as a way of strengthening the hand of local groups in their negotiations with decision-makers, indigenous involvement may be an important factor in the long-term objective of encouraging tenants to articulate their needs, and preparing them for their negotiations.

Of course, to do this, the survey must be seen as a matter of priority by the tenants. One Project worker, wishing to carry out a survey of the level of health care in a homeless-family block, found that the tenants' association was reluctant to help carry out the survey because they were engaged in negotiations with the Housing Department on the closure of the block. But if local people are involved in a survey this may impress the decision-makers with whom the group is to negotiate. There are, besides the matter of indigenous involvement, other problems inherent in using the survey method as a technique in community work practice which we shall explore in the following section.

The Survey Method as a Technique of Intervention

In community work the survey technique is sometimes used as a tool to legitimate the action of the community worker, or of community groups when they present their claims and needs to decision-makers. Official bodies are not easily persuaded when attempts to change them are not backed up by evidence.

The 'facts' produced by survey approaches can give a community group negotiating strength in bargaining that may take place. Impressions about the felt needs of a community are often vague, even though they are widely shared and acknowledged. On the other hand, the collection and careful analysis of facts is problematic and filled with traps for the community worker. First, there are the practical problems. Often, the community worker will have only limited technical and theoretical knowledge of survey techniques with which to make decisions about the type, size and extent of the survey. He will have to deal with questions of cost in terms of time, people and other resources to conduct the survey. He must ensure that questions are relevant, comprehensible, and not open to more than one interpretation. He must plan for a pre-test of the questionnaire to correct errors in order to avoid incomprehensible questions and inappropriate length. Finally, he will require the time and expertise that are necessary to correlate and analyse findings so that they can be interpreted to the group and to others. These initial considerations require an understanding of the tentative nature of the findings of such surveys. He must be able to understand whether the data support and validate his impressions or deny and confound the impressions of needs, and to recognise new issues previously not considered that may be revealed by the data. Thus, the survey is a piece of time-consuming work that is often regarded as an important weapon in building up knowledge in the community and providing ammunition but which may in fact fail to produce intended results. The constraints of objectivity and fairness must be balanced against other goals if the worker's credibility is to be maintained.

The consumer survey may be used by the community worker not only as a means of influence or to provide groups with ammunition. It is a means of entry into a community, a means of encouraging people to talk with each other about common concerns. It is also useful in focusing discussion around common problems and issues.

Finally, the technique may have negative consequences. For

example, the generation of the expectation of action to follow from such activities may lead to disillusionment about community organising if the survey results do not lead to action.

We have given a good deal of attention to the use of the survey because it is, along with the petition, one of the most commonly used methods of community work intervention. There are, of course, others that are more informal and unstructured. A worker may make contact with residents by intervening in a situation where residents have attempted to get together as consumers of a local service. For instance, he might make contact with parents of a local playgroup. Besides the fact that this kind of setting provides easy access to information and informal relationships, there are some sound practice principles for intervening at this level.

If the network of informal social life and contacts (which has its interstices in places like the local playgroup) supports sustained and effective formal neighbourhood organisations, the worker may find it is useful first to gain acceptance and credibility in these informal settings. For example, Project records describe several occasions on which Project workers intervened in the life of an estate by contacting mothers at local playgroups. For instance, a Project worker who had found it difficult to establish contact with tenants eventually discovered that several mothers from the estate went to a local playgroup whose leader was already known to the worker. The worker spent several afternoons hanging around the playgroup helping with the children and endeavouring to chat, though not very successfully, with the mothers. One afternoon the playgroup leader suggested a kind of informal tea party with the mothers when they came to collect their children. At the party the worker was given the opportunity to say something about himself and his work and to ask the mothers if there were any problems with which he could help. After several meetings it was decided to hold a Christmas party, and the worker and a small group of mothers worked for several weeks organising and carrying out plans for the party.

It was through the successful organisation of the party that the mothers learnt to know the worker and his objectives. They also acquired some beginning confidence in their ability to plan and work together. In addition, preparing for the party had increased the worker's knowledge about the estate and his acquaintance with other residents through his participation in advertising the Christmas party by leaflet.

Another mode of intervention used by the Project was to write to residents through the mail. For example, the Project wrote to residents in two blocks on one estate. The tenants' association had asked the Project to help in obtaining residents' views about life on the estate in order to strengthen its ability to negotiate with housing management. A letter was sent to residents asking if the worker could visit and talk with them on a certain day, inviting them to telephone if they did not want to be seen or would not be available on that date. This initial effort, like that which preceded the survey on the GLC post-war estate, softened the initial encounters between the residents and the investigating stranger; the initiative is left with the residents who are given the opportunity and time to consider whether they want to participate in such an exchange.

ORGANISING AROUND A SPECIFIC ISSUE

Goodwin Buildings was a slum block of some fifty flats built in the 1880s. It stood at the intersection of two busy main roads next to a row of four shops, two of which were open and two of which had been derelict for several years. In January 1972, a small notice was posted on two corners of the building, pasted up high on the wall so that vandals could not scrape it off. It was so high that it was almost impossible for a tall man to read comfortably. The notice, from the Department of the Environment, written in English that baffled most of the building's residents, advised of a public enquiry to be held at the Town Hall about the following matters:

the local authority's request to compulsorily purchase the building and shops and to use the site to provide open space; and
the local authority's failure to respond to a solicitor's request for planning permission to use one of the derelict shops for business purposes.

By chance, one of the Project workers saw the notice. The worker recorded that he approached a local playground leader and the secretary of a neighbouring tenants' association who was well known in Goodwin Buildings. It was decided to advertise the public enquiry in Goodwin by a leaflet. The worker was introduced by the playground leader to a liked and respected resident who helped him distribute the leaflets and draw up a petition that supported the

SOME OPENING MOVES IN NEIGHBOURHOOD WORK 85

compulsory purchase of the building. The local playground committee was enlisted to help collect signatures in the neighbourhood. A public meeting was called for the residents of the tenement by the local tenants' association, the local playground and by the individual residents who had helped in advertising and petition collection. The public meeting was held in a local club and a tenants' committee formed.

Our particular interest in these events is in the way in which the Department·of the Environment notice pasted on the sides of buildings served to define the issue for the worker, giving him a number of opportunities for intervention in the situation.

From the account of what followed we can identify a number of ways in which a worker can utilise an important event or a decision that may affect the well-being of a group to approach residents or extant organisations. The worker considers how to introduce himself to the local community and decides whether the concerns and auspices of his agency will make sense to, or alienate, the people to whom he talks. He also has to provide some explanation of why he is interested in the particular issue about which he is approaching residents. There may also emerge a conflict between the worker's own interests in the issue and those of the residents. For instance, another Project worker recorded:

'It became evident that the feelings of the tenants were not directly in line with the aims of the community group nor indeed with my own. I had gone on to the estate with various assumptions about how tenants might react to the redevelopment issue. Had they all wished to stay on this estate, this would have provided the group with good ammunition against the council and myself with possibly interesting and satisfying work. It was necessary, however, to re-appraise the situation when I found out that many of the tenants in fact wanted to leave the estate and the area. I had to become aware of how much my involvement would be detrimental to this group of residents. For those who wanted to stay I had possibly already raised expectations which I would be unable to fulfil, and this had to be made clear to other residents; it was necessary that any contact be constructive for them also; not, for example, to work purely with those tenants who wanted to stay and, therefore, work against the interests of a group of tenants who expressed very strongly their desire to leave the estate.'

In this case the worker dealt with the problem by assuming the role of information-giver; she supplied all tenants with as much data as possible about the redevelopment and demolition of the estate and spelled out the implications this could have for them. A news sheet, distributed to all tenants, gave details of the plan. This was followed up by a small information session in the yard of the estate. The worker was assisted at this session by some of the tenants who had been contacted earlier.

The Use of Petitions

The petition is a form of intervention that is frequently used by community groups. The petition serves a number of purposes: it conveys views to decision-makers about the issues in question; it spreads information in the locality about the issues; and it helps to recruit interested people and provides a way into the neighbourhood for the worker. Likewise, the residents' group who draw up the petition acquire new ideas, information and encouragement from those whom they ask to sign the petition. A well-supported petition is also useful in attracting media coverage which helps to consolidate the value of the petition in spreading knowledge and winning neighbourhood support. The expression of support contained in a petition is also useful in encouraging those local people who may be concerned about an issue but who are diffident in taking an activist role in organisations.

Public Meetings

When the issues have been defined in advance, the worker will be concerned with helping to form a group around the issue, or strengthening an extant group perhaps by passing on to it information that it may not have. Accounts of the Project experience reveal some of the painstaking ways by which workers made contact with residents on an individual basis before moving with them to the stage of committee meeting or steering group, and then to the next stage of public meeting. In our view, the public meeting should be considered as the outcome of preliminary efforts at intervention by the community worker rather than as a mechanism that is useful by itself as a way of identifying and recruiting members to its work. Of course, in many instances workers successfully take the initiative in distributing leaflets in a block or estate, inviting residents to a public meeting to discuss issues of concern. The outcome depends, obviously, on whether the worker has made appropriate judgements about the area and the issues facing its residents. We suspect, however, that the probabilities of success in using a public meeting as the initial means of contact are not great.

If we look more closely at the account of the worker who formed an adventure playground association with local residents we find that the process went something like this: as a result of her talks with some of the people in the area, the worker discovered their concern about play space. She made contact with a local curate and the tenants' associations on the issue of play. The people she contacted met with the worker to devise a strategy for sounding out neighbourhood views. A petition was circulated on a Sunday morning and over a thousand signatures were collected. The group saw themselves as a steering group and arranged for the petition to be presented to the local authority. During the petitioning of the area, they reported:

'We had told people that we would be calling a public meeting shortly to elect a committee and that we would let them know when this takes place. We agreed that we should hold a meeting prior to that to plan it and that we should invite others to the meeting; not only those involved so far but people who had shown an especial interest when we had called upon them.'

A steering group then met to plan a public meeting and design leaflets and posters to advertise it, and subsequent meetings were held to put up posters and deliver leaflets. During this activity, knowledge and interest in the issue of play and in the forthcoming meeting was fostered in the neighbourhood information network. Slides of different kinds of playgrounds were shown, and the committee was elected for the year. Some five months elapsed between the time the worker latched on to the issue of play and the public meeting to elect a committee.

Without this kind of care and planning the public meeting can be a hazardous form of intervention. It can be a problematic form of intervention for other reasons. In choosing tenants to attend a meeting, the worker or a group-in-embryo can invite everyone to the meeting in order to see who turns up, in effect allowing individuals themselves to decide whether they will attend. On the other hand, the worker can retain control of attendance by inviting only tenants he has 'selected' on certain criteria. The worker who intervened in a post-war GLC estate, for instance, argued that a small group of highly motivated residents would stand a better chance of successfully organising themselves. He was also conscious that calling a public meeting would alienate the members of the established social club. There are, too, practical grounds for the community worker to avoid calling a public meeting. He may be aware, for instance, that few residents are likely to turn out to a meeting in response to a printed leaflet shoved through their letter-box. A better strategy would be for the worker to visit each person on the estate personally, inviting them to come to the public meeting and giving them the chance to question the worker about the purpose of the meeting and be reassured by him that other tenants would be coming. People are unlikely to come to a meeting if they feel they may stand the risk of looking foolish when it is found that no one else came. A public meeting requires that tenants make an overt display of interest and concern for an issue. They may be more disposed to make such a public commitment if the worker, or an embryonic group, has promoted discussion and knowledge of the issue around the estate. Likewise, the worker may have doubts about support for the views and leadership claims of people who too readily assert themselves in large groups. A worker who calls to a public meeting tenants with whom he has had little previous involvement emphasises that he is a stranger; moreover, if the tenants are strangers to one another, they may look to the worker for initiative in setting the agenda for, and organising, the meeting. The community worker may feel that such a high profile role is inappropriate. The public meeting as a way of initially organising and recruiting tenants may satisfy the worker's need for 'action' but may do little to help tenants learn more about the issue and the worker, and about the ramifications of their involvement in organised collective action.

Chapter 5

A COALITION: THE RESIDENTS

We have indicated that the Project was not in business to provide a casework service in the community; in respect of its neighbourhood activities is was concerned with assisting groups to articulate their needs and objectives and take collective action on them. Understanding the relationship between a community resource like the Project and community residents requires that we examine the relationships between a worker and a group that are implied by phrases like 'concerned with groups' or 'assisting groups'. Understanding these ideas may help us better to understand the links between neighbourhood resources and the people who live and work in the community, and the factors that facilitate and hinder the achievement of community work goals.

We start by describing the relationship between a community work project and user groups as a *coalition* attempting to act as another community resource. By *coalition* we mean the *temporary alliance of distinct parties for a limited purpose.*[1]

The relationship between a project and its users is *temporary* for a number of reasons. Funds are available for a limited period only. The members of a project team are not committed to remain in the neighbourhood, as many residents are. Indeed, only one of the workers appointed at the start of the SCP, for instance, remained to the end of the Project. There is another sense in which the relationship is temporary: that is, project team members do not, usually, live in the area and team members withdraw from the neighbourhood at the end of their day and week. The alliance is also interrupted by staff holidays. For example, team members at the SCP were entitled to seven weeks annual leave; and, of course, work at the SCP was interrupted by teaching and other commitments at the Institute. Moreover, from the point of view of a user group, the relationship is temporary not just because people have other commitments such as earning a living and bringing up a family but because the alliance is dissolved when the group's aims

[1] Taken from *The Shorter Oxford English Dictionary*, third edition, 1964.

are achieved. In the case of slum clearance, members of groups may move out of the area altogether. (However, there were several participants in north-west Southwark who continued to use the area socially after they had moved and who helped nascent community groups with similar objectives.)

The relationship between a community development project and its users is, in part, affected by the wide-ranging objectives of community groups. Some groups may be concerned with the clearance and demolition of slum housing while others are working on the provision and management of an adventure playground; some groups may focus on extracting benefits for the community from a proposed redevelopment of the neighbourhood. But from the point of view of each group these purposes are parochial and limited by the degree of success in solving a local problem, though the work of some groups (e.g. on redevelopment and homeless families) may have far-reaching implications. The purpose of this kind of collective action is limited not only to the problems facing localities but also to those problems amenable to solution by exerting pressure at a local or borough-wide level.

The several parties or interests in the coalitive structure are normally distinct in respect of their values, socio-economic realities, family situation and life style, nationality, age, sex, and political ideologies and commitments. The workers, on the one hand, are often products of the universities of an educational system that has discriminated against those brought up in the neighbourhood. The community workers earn comparatively large salaries and enjoy other privileges such as long holidays that can affect the relationship of the workers to the neighbourhood groups. The workers' holidays can cause anxiety to some group members if they have not become secure in their own capacity. The worker may be seen as a dilettante who is not always available when needed.

The users of a project, on the other hand, will form an equally distinct interest in that they are tied to neighbourhood and class by virtue of residence, work and their limited training and experience. But there are often differences among the user groups themselves and the individual participants.

We begin this analysis of the alliances that constitute the coalitive structure by looking at the relationships that may develop between the user groups; following that we will examine the contribution that users make to the coalition.

RELATIONSHIPS AMONG USERS

We refer here only to users who are neighbourhood groups or residents. Work with service agencies will be discussed in a later chapter.

We have noted that neighbourhood groups who used the SCP were, with two major exceptions, resident within a quarter of a mile of the Project base and that the catchment area for work with individuals who used the Project was less than 200 yards from the Project door.

Many neighbourhood projects have found that the closer groups and individuals are (geographically) to a resource the more likely they are to use its services. A community work project meets the administrative needs of groups and provides them with a place to meet. Both these services must be near to the people concerned in order to encourage attendance at meetings and to enable committee members to use them when commitments to families and jobs allow. When they are beginning, most neighbourhood projects are unknown commodities to local people. Therefore, the use of services relies on effective practice in the field situation and on dissemination of information about the services through the neighbourhood news and gossip networks. If these networks are small and limited, they will result in a limited catchment area for the project. This also accounts in part for the difficulty that community work projects experience in being selective about the quantity and kind of work they attract. It is difficult to refuse the services of a project to any group of local residents because the effectiveness of neighbourhood information networks will assure that such a refusal will be made known to other groups and possibly inhibit people from using the project.

One of the consequences of the proximity of groups in the limited catchment area of the SCP was that the team members were able to maintain weekly, often daily, contact with most user groups. This continuous contact enabled group members to come to the Project during the day, in a lunch break, or whilst shopping, so that they carried out the work of the group and made contacts with other groups, students and service agency personnel; they also learned to take responsibility for answering the Project telephone and to help with enquiries off the street about social security, housing problems, and so forth. A further consequence of proximity for the SCP staff was that they made deliberate efforts to help residents who lived within the Project target area but outside its catchment area. The SCP also worked closely with community workers in other parts of the borough, maintaining borough-wide contacts by circulating papers on common issues and attending committees and conferences.

The size of the catchment area is one of the factors that determines the relationships among users of a project. Neighbourhood groups in small catchment areas are more likely to learn about one another's concerns. In north-west Southwark, the neighbourhood groups were, on the whole, bound together by their common residence in inadequate housing provision and their shared experience of poor resources in the neighbourhood. Not only were they neighbours but most were in negotiation with the Greater London Council and the London Borough of Southwark. Co-operation and friendship developed among these groups and they often sought advice and encouragement from one another. There was among the groups a league of merit; groups that were concerned with slum clearance tended to be scornful of people concerned with what they thought to be unimportant issues like estate maintenance, welfare and recreational facilities.

Competition for Resources

Groups compete with one another for the scarce resources of a neighbourhood. For instance, two or three tenants' associations simultaneously attempting to achieve the rehousing of people from their blocks were competing for the comparatively scarce housing units of the local authority and the Greater London Council. On several occasions residents who had been in slum housing for most of their lives were resentful at the apparent efficiency of the tenants' association of a neighbouring block for homeless families in effecting the rehousing of its constituents. They spoke about the fecklessness and queue-jumping proclivities of homeless families:

'People seemed generally very cross that the Curate had been sticking up for tenants in the homeless family block whom they considered to be all immoral and dirty and who didn't deserve housing, and if they got housing first would be housed in front of respectable tenants like themselves who had been in the area a great deal longer and had worse housing conditions.'

One time, a local tenants' chairman arranged a tour of his

nineteenth-century slum for the chairman and officers of the home-less families' association who were appalled at the state of accom-modation in the slum but none the less resolute in their attempts to help families escape not just from the poor standard of homeless family accommodation but also from its stigma.

Groups also compete for the resources of a community project. If the project is so responsive a resource that project staff never decline to give help to a local group, the staff may find that they are simply giving an increasingly diluted service to the groups using the project. Therefore, it is useful to have an agency policy about what kinds of groups might claim priority in the use of project staff and services. Over-commitment of the time and energy of the team members will negate their being available at appropriate times to work with groups. Faced with two or three group meet-ings on one evening, the worker has to decide which to attend. In the absence of agency criteria for making this decision, the worker must decide for himself and his decisions might not be in the project's larger interest.

There will also be competition amongst groups, and between groups and staff for the use of rooms and secretarial services. The secretaries in the SCP had to make their own decisions about which group's work was done first, and whether work from a staff mem-ber took precedence over work for a group. Groups varied, of course, in the demands they made upon the SCP, but 'heavy users' like Chaucer House and the North Southwark Community Development Group were often criticised for the amount of staff time and other resources that they utilised. In these circumstances, groups joked that a worker was a particular chairman's 'private secretary' and that the worker could be seen 'by appointment only'.

On a few occasions in the work of the SCP, the officers of groups attended meetings of other neighbourhood groups. Such inter-group activity took place towards the last year of the Project and only in relation to issues common to the neighbourhood such as the quality of the service provided by the social services department. Officers seldom went with one another to meetings with the local authority or other parts of officialdom.

Community workers act as mediators between the groups who use a project. SCP staff had to deal with concerns about some groups and individuals who used the Project as a refuge from bad housing conditions or unhappy marital situations. One group was

94   ORGANISING FOR SOCIAL CHANGE

extremely reluctant to use the Project, except for evening meetings, because they thought it had been taken over by the homeless families tenants' association. Workers were frequently invited to join in 'gossip' about other groups, particularly by members of newly-formed groups who wished to match their progress against more experienced community groups. Residents often wanted to talk about the development of other groups, and how they tackled problems like maintaining interest and attracting new members, handling finance and coping with maverick members. The question asked most frequently about other groups was in regard to the numbers present at meetings. SCP workers were careful in responding to questions of this kind, not wishing to appear judgemental about the functioning of groups. Sometimes such questions were a means of introducing discussion on a personal or a group problem rather than real interest in the other group; sometimes the discussion was initiated to boost confidence after a setback in the group's work such as an unsatisfactory meeting; but as often these questions were an attempt to confirm that the worker was interested in the group, particularly if he had been giving more time to other users of the Project.

A project provides a base and a number of facilities that a variety of groups use in common. This inter-group activity is important in giving confidence, skills and knowledge to many individuals belonging to groups, and it presents opportunities for inter-group learning.

THE CONTRIBUTION OF NEIGHBOURHOOD GROUPS

When we seek change through community action we imply that organisations (e.g. the local authority, the GLC, and housing trusts) and individuals (e.g. private landlords) who control resources relevant to a locality like north-west Southwark are less able to resist pressures for change when they are exerted by organisations of residents rather than individuals. The range of negotiating techniques and strategies available to an individual in a deprived neighbourhood is generally weak because organisations can withstand or absorb or deflect individuals acting as change agents either on behalf of themselves or their friends or even on behalf of their neighbours as a whole. Of course, individuals are not altogether powerless. The effectiveness of individual attempts at change depends in part on the magnitude of the desired change. One

Project worker, for instance, wrote of an occasion when one of the long-established residents in the area came to the Project complaining that the dustbins in her block had not been emptied for a week:

'I did not accede to her request that I telephone the council and "get them to do something about it". Rather, I gave her the telephone, the number to ring and the name of the man responsible for queries about refuse collection. The poor man did not know what hit him, and she weighed into him with an uninterrupted flow of curses, blasphemies and invective on the inability of bureaucrats to get up from their seats. The bins in the block were emptied that afternoon.'

The Project attempted to transform the attempts of individuals into group efforts to seek collective solutions to problems. There were many instances of failure of individuals to achieve change in respect of resources. This is what one Project worker wrote of a tenants' association meeting:

'The steering committee met with more than a dozen participants from all over the estate. A number of people in the group reported recent efforts they had made as individuals to get improvements on the estate which had all failed to get action taken. For example, one man had written letters to the District Housing Manager about the effects of revamping one of the blocks on the estate. . . . No one was surprised to hear that he had received no reply. The general view was that an association of some kind might be regarded as carrying more weight than individual complaints.'

The worker's record indicates that no tenant was surprised that the man did not receive a reply to his letters. They were accustomed to the idea and some even accepted it as natural and inevitable that they would be treated rudely by Housing Department officials. The futility and frustration of individual pestering of organisations is best illustrated by the experiences of a local resident. After the Department of the Environment had refused the GLC a compulsory order to close his block, he spent considerable time and effort in finding out what would happen to the residents:

'I couldn't get a straight answer from anyone. They are all putter-offers up there – they keep putting you off, sending you

from one department to another. Eventually, I took a week off
work just to sort out what was going to happen to us. I went to
County Hall and they said it was out of their hands, and sent
me to see the council. The housing people sent me to see the
Health, and they told me to go back to the GLC. I spent the
whole week going from one person to another, and I never got
the information I wanted. They just kept putting me off, putting
me off. . . .'

A few weeks after a tenants' association was formed in this
block, they visited the chairman of the GLC Housing Committee,
their GLC councillor and the local MP and obtained the information they wanted. Subsequently, they were put in touch with the
housing association who had been negotiating for some time to buy
the block for improvement.

The Strengths of Collective Action

The strength of neighbourhood groups is twofold: first is the support, encouragement and invulnerability that a group offers to its
members. Collective action provides support for individual efforts
to achieve change and its relative anonymity encourages individuals
to act. Encouragement and support from the group helps residents
to take up more public roles as officers of committees. Likewise,
the group provides a buttress for residents who take prominent
negotiating roles. A further strength of collective action is that it
provides a learning situation where inter-personal skills are
acquired that are relevant to a person's ability in negotiations with
resource decision-makers.

The second strength of neighbourhood groups is the range of
negotiating techniques open to them. Neighbourhood groups
usually begin negotiations by using letters, telephone calls, and
personal visits to seek relevant information regarding changes the
group desires. A worker may encourage involvement at this level
of negotiation to ensure that the group acquires cohesion, skills and
self-confidence. Inevitably, frustration and anger increase as the
limited usefulness of these modes of negotiation become manifest
and the group will turn to negotiating with resource decision-
makers by petition, deputation, demonstration, rent strike, court
action, and by harnessing the pressure which skilful publicity can
exert. Organisations and individuals who control or make decisions

about community resources are quite vulnerable to publicity about the plight of the group, particularly when it highlights the inadequate response of the resource decision-makers to the group.

1 *The use of the media.* The presence and support of the television and local and national Press is crucial to many collective forms of organised protest. The skilful use of the media can strengthen a neighbourhood group's hand in negotiations. Local authority departments are particularly vulnerable to adverse publicity about any shortfalls or inadequacies in the services they provide. Coverage of a group's activities in the local and national media can engender public support for the group, and spread knowledge about its work and its objectives. Local groups in Southwark came to know which television programmes and newspapers were likely to give sympathetic attention to their campaigns. On television, the programmes 'Today', 'Nationwide' and 'Man Alive' were highly regarded for the help they gave to the efforts of neighbourhood action groups; many groups sought and found, sometimes helpful, sometimes adverse, publicity in the *South London Press*, and occasionally in the *Evening Standard* but rarely in one of the national papers, although the *Daily Telegraph*, the *Guardian* and the *City News* have carried features about the work of some groups in north-west Southwark.

The group in north-west Southwark that received the most consistent and widespread media coverage was the Chaucer House Tenants' Association, whose committee developed considerable expertise in using the media to expose and embarrass the London Borough of Southwark and its policy for housing homeless families. The BBC made a ninety-minute documentary on the committee's work which was broadcast in September and December 1972 to the entire country. The barricading of social workers and housing officials from their offices in Chaucer House and the bonfires of uncollected refuse would have had limited impact without the media coverage of the protest which clarified the objectives of the tenants' association.

The committee was often charged by the council and other detractors with 'organising demonstrations for the benefit of the TV cameras'. But in their view they did not exploit the media for vainglorious reasons or to acquire prestige or notoriety. They tended to be circumspect in dealings with the media because they wished to avoid pejorative presentations of tenants. Some tenants objected to the publicity on the grounds that it embarrassed them at work or within their families.

The use of the media enabled the Chaucer House committee to stimulate tenants who might otherwise have been resigned to bad housing and apathetic about the work of the committee. The presence of television cameras at the committee's Annual General Meeting ensured an unprecedented attendance. Tenants may have come in order to see themselves later on television, but they participated in the meeting and increased their knowledge of the committee and its work. There is nothing disreputable in this; indeed, one of the central points of experiments in community television and video tape techniques is the effect of self-presentation before a camera (and subsequent play-back) on generating people's enthusiasms and interests in community affairs. Video has been successfully used to break down people's apathy and lack of involvement in community issues.

Exploitation of the media will lead to misunderstandings about the role of community workers by public agencies who are frequently the objects of public scrutiny. It will often be believed that the community workers are 'behind it all', or that 'they put the group up to it'. This was the case during Southwark's negotiations with the squatters and, later, with the Chaucer House Tenants' Association. The following is a Project worker's report of a telephone conversation with Southwark's public relations department:

'Mr X came on to the phone and . . . a long and somewhat confused conversation about the press conference followed, together with his and the council's reaction to "The Block", the BBC documentary on Chaucer House. . . . He went on for a considerable time with comments about the documentary, feeling that the main issue of social deprivation was lost because of the emotive handling of the facts. All this was inter-linked with innuendoes about the Project's role and that these events had set back progress being made "elsewhere". It was difficult for me to sort out when he was talking about the redevelopment group's recent publicity and the attack on the strategy plan, and when he was talking about "The Block" and its consequences. It was apparent that both had impact and were being attributed by officers in the London Borough of Southwark to the hidden hand of the Project. I said that a similar sort of scapegoating of the Project had occurred after the arrival of the squatters in Southwark.'

The Project's contribution to the making of 'The Block' was extremely limited; the team declined an invitation from the press officer to attend a meeting at the Town Hall with the producer of the documentary and refused to participate or appear in the film. They had collaborated only to the extent of making the producer welcome at the Project and inviting him to use material it might have on the borough and on the situation of homeless families.

The report of the telephone conversation with the public relations department also refers to a press conference held by the North Southwark Community Development Group to release its criticisms of the local authority's draft strategy plan for redevelopment in north-west Southwark. The department's misunderstanding of the role of the community group in the press conference was shared by many members of the council's planning department who saw the conference as an unnecessary and hostile act on the part of the group. The following are the values the press conference had for the group:

it ensured that the group's comments would not be ignored as the comments of the previous critics of the plans had been;
press coverage ensured that local residents and workers had an additional source of information about the group's work; it helped to allay fears they might have that nothing was being done to oppose redevelopment plans that threatened their homes and jobs;
the press coverage encouraged group members in their work; it was a tangible achievement, important when the work of the group was concerned with complex, long-term issues;
the sympathetic response from the Press served to strengthen the confidence of group members; it provided validation that they were right to be critical about the redevelopment plans;
the publicity established contacts with other groups of residents concerned with redevelopment issues elsewhere in London; several professionals and students offered volunteer services to help the group as a result;
good press coverage stimulated the interest of the television companies; the group's work was not only covered by television,

but it produced income for the group which it needed to finance its day-to-day operations. (In north-west Southwark several groups learned to insist on fees for appearing on television or giving lectures and seminars.)

When appropriate, it is incumbent upon groups to attract as much media coverage as is possible because the dissemination of information may be helpful to other groups negotiating similar issues. In addition, the group's activities may act as a catalyst for unorganised residents facing similar issues and/or groups looking for more effective strategies or modes of organisation.

2 *Exploiting rivalries.* Resource decision-makers are vulnerable to other forms of manipulation and coercion by neighbourhood groups. For instance, the sympathy of elected members with the objectives of a neighbourhood group may be greater if the elected member's political position is more marginal. Politicians of minority parties seeking votes may also be more likely than others to respond to the interests of groups. This was not the case for groups in north-west Southwark, however, because the Labour Party had been returned there for many years without serious opposition. There was no necessity, therefore, for the elected member to secure votes by courting the favour of neighbourhood groups. Nevertheless, many groups were able to exert pressure on councillors and officials by other strategies. For instance, rivalries and animosities between different chief officers and departments could be exploited; groups often found field workers in departments more sympathetic and helpful than middle and senior management, especially when groups supported field staff in policy disputes with their seniors; chairmen of committees were kept informed of negotiations at officer level, and the support of local Members of Parliament was often sought in negotiations with the local authority.

Inter- and intra-organisational tensions and competitiveness can be exploited by local groups to strengthen their position in negotiations with decision-makers. For example, in Southwark some neighbourhood groups exploited the rivalry between the entrenched, older paternalistic councillors from the former Metropolitan boroughs of Southwark and Bermondsey, and the councillors from Dulwich and Camberwell who were a younger, more progressive, professional, house-owning population.

3 *Attraction of human resources.* A successfully functioning group attracts a wide variety of resources, largely in the form of student and professional volunteer help, which can provide many skills relevant to the group's negotiations with organisations. Thus several of the tenants' associations in north-west Southwark had access to the free advice of lawyers, surveyors, architects and planners. The playground committee recruited surveyors and architects to help them plan the site and a variety of students interested in working with children. The North Southwark Community Development Group (NSCDG) attracted planners, geographers, sociologists, architects, and a local historian who carried out research tasks on its behalf. These professionals and student resources supplemented and enhanced the work of NSCDG, and learning to use resources of this kind was important in the development of the Group. There were several occasions when students and professionals descended on NSCDG to help 'save' north-west Southwark, and they were politely told to go back where they came from; yet there were many others who, by the diligence of their work for the Group and the manner in which they built relationships of trust and understanding with members, made a valuable contribution to all levels of the Group's activities. On the whole, these were people who lived in or near north-west Southwark, who not only had a locus as residents, but who had also acquired a feeling for the neighbourhood and the activities of the Group.

4 *Attracting finance.* Neighbourhood groups are often success-ful in raising substantial sums of money to pursue their interests and employ their own workers. Groups also acquire resources in kind. The Mint Street Adventure Playground Association, for instance, received help from local residents in clearing and pre-paring a site, and making equipment for the playground and play hut. Several local firms were generous to some groups by donating paper, writing and painting materials, and food and drink for events like jumble sales and fairs.

5 *Facilitating public participation.* Organised community action facilitates discussion and negotiation between organisations like the local authority and local residents on neighbourhood issues that are broader than the concerns of any particular community group. An appendix to the Hornsey plan of the Association of

Neighbourhood Councils stated it this way: 'Apart from the advantage to local people, the assistance of such machinery [neighbourhood councils] would clearly be a great help to local elected representatives anxious to consult and co-operate with local opinion, and indeed to local authorities themselves.'

This sentiment was endorsed by the Greater London Council Housing Committee in its report on the public participation programme in the Swinbrooke Road area of Notting Hill. The report said:

'With the presence of the neighbourhood council, development work had been carried out in advance to organise people and make them aware of issues . . . the local community was organised into its own committees, was aware of issues in advance, could give useful ideas and could cope with the situation that in other areas might have been overwhelming.'

In north-west Southwark, the organisation of the community into groups facilitated discussion with the local authority and GLC on a number of issues: chairmen of tenants' associations met with the area team of the social services department; residents were represented on the Rockingham Estate Multi-Service Group; the Rockingham Estate Community and the Rockingham Adventure Playground were represented on the study group planning for the multi-service centre and community hall; the NSCDG and the local authority met in negotiation on the redevelopment of north Southwark.

The Costs and Benefits of Collective Action

The successful functioning of a coalition of project workers and neighbourhood users results in costs and benefits to residents. Those who serve on committees acquire prestige and status among their peers; they also may increase their knowledge and skills, and gain satisfaction in helping materially to improve the well-being of the community. Some residents attributed improvements in their jobs to skills and confidence gained through community action. Women active in neighbourhood groups frequently expressed their awareness of their increased competence and capacity to undertake previously unimagined leadership roles. We have already noted in Chapter 1 the strength of women in the internal support network of the neighbourhood. Involvement in community action seems to have emancipated many working-class women in north-west

Southwark who acquired positions of strength in the neighbour-hood as well as in the home.

On the other hand, participation in community action demands a great deal of those who take committee and officer roles; for instance, the health of one or two chairmen of groups in north-west Southwark was threatened by the amount of time and energy they gave to their work. There is, too, a great deal of self- and family-sacrifice, particularly amongst officers of tenants' associa-tions. Officers are 'on call' for virtually twenty-four hours a day to cope with individual problems concerning housing, social security, police and a variety of other matters.

Participants find it exhausting and spouses find it irritating when they are constantly coping with the stress and difficulties ex-perienced by their neighbours. The commitment of officers to the work of a group often provokes criticism and resentment from spouses. Not only are husbands less available to help with family chores and activities like shopping and taking holidays, but their wives are, on the whole, not involved in the work of the group. The husband's concern with 'important business' might threaten spouses who fear that the husband's experiences will create distance and tension between them. Some wives may feel that they and their families are being neglected because of the man's commit-ment to the work of his group. For instance, the wife of an officer of a tenants' association confided to a Project worker: 'He spends all his time in helping other people, but he does nothing for me and the family. We never see him, he never takes us out anywhere. He is not a real husband any more.' Another worker, asked by some husbands about how his wife felt when he was out so often in the evenings, wrote the following:

'I used to reply that my wife understood the work I did and I always tried to keep her informed of it, and involve her as much as possible. M said: "My wife's grumbling like mad that she doesn't see me any more. I'm going to give her hard times one of these days to shut her up." I said that would not be fair, after all, she is missing you, she is stuck in one room all day, and you can escape from it by coming down to the Project to work. You might like to bring her down with you – Joy needs some help with the filing – and try to keep her informed of the work you are doing and allay her fears that your rehousing will be held up because of your work with the tenants' group.'

Of course, husbands may be resentful when their wives take prominent roles in neighbourhood groups. We found a large degree of conservatism in north-west Southwark about women assuming leadership roles; many people felt that there was something not quite right about women going out for the evenings alone to attend meetings. On several occasions, husbands were clearly suspicious that meetings were being used as opportunities to carry on extra-marital liaisons. The following report is a good illustration:

'Halfway through the meeting, Mary made a sign that Jack was outside and would I leave the meeting to talk to him. I went outside and Jack was furious at Mary being filmed by TV cameras, and also because several of the male committee members were telephoning her at work. We marched up and down the pavement in the bitter cold while he threatened to go in and drag her out. He eventually relented and insisted that Mary not stand for re-election. I took him home and promised to take Mary home by car. Mary nevertheless stood and was re-elected, saying "There'll be hell to pay tonight . . ." In the event, Jack prevented her coming to committee meetings by going out with his mates on Monday nights so she had to stay home to look after the children.'

Residents may find that their involvement with neighbourhood groups is costly financially. Attendance at evening meetings, for instance, robs men and women of the opportunity of overtime or casual evening jobs. In addition, committee members may lose a morning's or an afternoon's wages in order to prosecute the group's work, attending a meeting, or accompanying a constituent to the social security offices. Husbands may give up work opportunities in the evenings to look after children while their wives attend meetings. Committee members incur expenses of travelling and telephone calls made on behalf of the group. At one hectic stage in the life of a tenants' association, several officers remained unemployed in order to push forward the interest of the group which required their availability during the day. The Department of Health and Social Security enabled, albeit unwittingly, several local people to become more or less full-time workers for their groups. Many residents found it difficult to escape from the number of demands made on their time and energies by community action. Not only did residents have to cope with the interests of their own group, but they were often asked to help new groups, to speak at meetings and to attend borough-wide meetings. Residents struggled with the problems of earning a living and raising a family and also had the worry and strain of running a committee, raising funds, employing workers, and dealing with all the crises and complaints that seem to be the natural consequence of community action programmes.

Participation in neighbourhood work also involves community members in a diversity of new, often bewildering experiences. Residents frequently find themselves in situations of stress such as meeting the chairman of a local authority committee or the local MP, chairing or speaking to a public meeting, talking to the Press, appearing on television, asking for funds in the august boardroom of a charitable foundation, speaking to students and social workers at a conference or a seminar, and representing constitutents at appeal tribunals.

Committee members are often acting on the margins of a culture which is not their own. In north-west Southwark, many found the long, gradual process of acculturation exhausting and nerve-racking; but many succeeded in pushing the boundary of what they considered to be impossible in terms of their own ability and confidence. These new experiences, as well as contact with professionals in a variety of situations, created tensions for at least two residents active in local groups who were simultaneously attracted to a middle-class style of life, embittered by its values, and rooted firmly in a working-class community by virtue of their educational background and employment.

SCP workers found that there were times when considerable animosity from constituents was directed against officers or groups. In at least two tenants' associations, principal officers were singled out both for private and public attack during the clearance of slum blocks. Several tenants felt resentful at not being amongst the first to be rehoused, and those who remained until last seemed to transfer their grievances with the rehousing authority to the leaders of the tenants' association, some of whom had already been rehoused.

Criticism of tenants' association officers was continually voiced. For instance, many residents in Chaucer House disagreed with the tactics of the committee which attracted publicity to those living in the block. It was all too easy in situations like this for officers of neighbourhood groups to be accused of 'publicity seeking'. There is no doubt that the prominence achieved by some chairmen created feelings of anger and envy among several constituents.

Feelings of animosity towards group leaders were particularly prevalent in tenant's associations concerned with clearing slum housing. The activities of a tenants' association may be seen by residents as a constant reproach to husbands of their failure to provide for their family, and the imagined reproach may be felt as strongly as the ethic that it is part of the man's responsibility to earn sufficient wages to provide a roof, food and clothing for his family. The success of the tenants' association, particularly where it is motivated by a group of charismatic figures, may be seen as emasculatory by the husbands in the slum. Tensions are created between constitutents and officers; and spouses will fear that their mate's activities in the association may conceal extra-marital liaisons; or the activities may painfully reveal that the male-female relationship in the committee situation is more satisfying than the one they have at home.

Chapter 6

A COALITION: THE COMMUNITY WORKER

We examine in this chapter the contribution of the community worker to the coalition of neighbourhood groups and the community work project.

THE ROLE OF THE COMMUNITY WORKER

The role of the community worker is often described in such terms as 'interpreter', 'communicator', 'enabler', 'facilitator', 'catalyst', and 'mediator'. Generally these are acceptable roles and from a public relations standpoint might be useful designations. They imply that the worker is objective regarding the content of decisions and action and that his role is to assist people to make decisions more efficiently by enabling them to understand all aspects of a situation.

No doubt, workers sometimes act this way but even at their most neutral they must decide whether to involve themselves in a situation and whether to remain with it; and, in order to enable and facilitate, they must continually assess situations and the consequences of various kinds of action; and, in the light of these judgements, they must decide how to intervene.

There are other designations of community worker roles that imply a more active stance for the worker such as 'stimulator', 'expeditor', 'negotiator', 'bargainer', 'advocate', 'expert' and 'planner'. Some of these terms imply a worker who assumes a more directive role regarding decisions and policies in community work. This more activist and partisan approach can be problematic. It may undermine the learning process, initiative and self-determination of other participants. It may antagonise participants who disagree with the worker. It places greater responsibility for the outcome of community action on the worker.

In practice, workers may adopt varying degrees of neutrality or activism depending upon what appears to be feasible and appropriate in particular situations. General principles that guide the approach of the worker must be utilised with an understanding of the content of inter-personal contacts implied by most of the roles mentioned above. What factors determine the relationship between the enabler and the enabled, between the stimulator and the stimulated, and between the advocate and those for whom he speaks?

Project Objectives

A major factor that determines the role of the community worker is the type of objectives of the project within which he works. For instance, the attempt to work with service agencies and to train students in the field situation limits the possible roles open to workers *vis-à-vis* neighbourhood groups by *limiting the choice of workers who might be employed in the project.* A concern with service agencies and with student placements means that the project staff will be likely to include well-educated and experienced professionals.

Time Frame

Another constraint on the worker's role is the time-limited nature of most community work intervention. Traditionally, community work projects have been established for periods of three to five years. Several problems should be anticipated when projects operate within narrow time limits: neighbourhood groups may not achieve their objectives within the project's time schedule; and a project will rarely meet the needs of all groups and residents within its comparatively brief intervention in the neighbourhood. Thus, the time-limited nature of a project will determine whether its workers will, to varying degrees, be as concerned with the organisational needs of groups as with the achievement of their goals in order that local people will continue to pursue their objectives after the community work project has left the area. Thus, a community work project that is established as a permanent feature of an area will afford workers a greater degree of choice in the roles they adopt as well as the opportunity to shift back and forth along the continuum of roles. It will be interesting, in this respect, to watch the development of permanent community work resources within the area teams of social services departments.

In a project of limited duration, the role of the community worker will be constrained by:

the temptation of wanting to achieve fairly tangible results in a short time. The groups using SCP, for instance, did not face up to the reality of SCP's withdrawal in January 1973 until May of the previous year. Given the desirability of attracting a new worker sufficiently early to provide an overlap of some three months with the outgoing workers, this left barely five months in which the Project users could come together and plan for a continuing community work resource in the area. This time proved insufficient and the groups were rushed through the process by the outgoing workers and did not understand fully what was happening. The workers' desire to leave behind a viable resource made them disregard the pace at which the groups were able to work;

the over-full timetables of community workers. This will reduce the amount of time, care and attention given to organisational skill development. Hence this may be neglected;

the incidence of staff turnover within a project: most projects can expect to experience some change of staffing, and new workers will be constrained in their roles by the expectations of community work intervention set for project users by the outgoing workers. Staff turnover reduces even further the amount of time that a worker can expect to give to local groups, and feelings of impatience and the temptation 'to get things done' may thus be aggravated;

the amount of time and contact a worker is likely to have with a group: we noted, for instance, several occasions in the work of SCP when community workers, present at meetings they would not normally expect to attend, adopted a more activist role;

the urgency of the neighbourhood group's objectives: if, for an example, a group discovers from a sympathetic councillor that the council intend to take a decision within a few days on a matter that affected the group, the worker will have to respond by doing things he might normally expect to leave to the group such as getting signatures to a petition, canvassing councillors, and contacting the Press.

THE PHASES OF A COMMUNITY WORKER'S INTERVENTION

The degree of activism of the worker varies with the phases of work with groups. Four phases in the development of a community group towards the achievement of its goals were identified in Chapter 1:

establishing an organisation;
identifying those who make decisions about resources;
developing skills and confidence within a group;
negotiating with those who make decisions about resources.

These phases in the life of a group are separated only for analytical purposes. It is not suggested that the phases are sequential. Indeed, we shall see that they might occur simultaneously.

Establishing an Organisation

In Chapter 4 we identified some of the ways in which a community worker achieves a working relationship with local residents. An already-formed group may come into the project to use its telephone or duplicator; an individual may come in with a personal problem in which the worker sees the opportunity for collective action; or the worker may discover groups of people with shared problems by actively seeking them out or by hanging about the neighbourhood.

The worker's role in the early stages of work is very active, not just in making contacts, but also in the advice he may give. Some individuals concerned with personal or local problems may be able to mobilise friends and neighbours to support collective action; others may see an issue only in personal terms (e.g. How can I get better housing?). Because of the worker's concern with collective action such individuals may be referred to another group or agency, or they might be advised to seek out neighbours with a similar problem in order to take collective action. In giving this advice the worker assumes a role of some authority. If the advice is accepted, the residents are launched on an enterprise the consequences of which they can hardly anticipate. It is an essential part of the worker's task to promote contact between novitiate residents and existing community groups so that anxieties are allayed and unrealistic expectations reduced, and to spell out the possible ramifications of collective action. Because residents may enter into collective action without a clear understanding, their decision represents an act of faith in a relatively unknown worker. This gives to the worker a higher degree of influence than he will have in later stages of a group's existence.

The worker's advice to take collective action requires that attention be given to the task of mobilising wider support for the issue and defining a structure and function for the group of residents. The worker and the nucleus of residents must decide on the following:

the initiative to choose (e.g. petition, survey, leaflet, personal calls);
how to share the work;
the best time for catching people in their flats;
the drafting of letters to accompany the petition, if any;
identifying those in authority to whom it will be sent.

The formation of a steering group is often the next phase of organisation for many groups. The functions of a steering group include planning and preparing the public meeting at which the group's committee will be elected. In the case of an adventure playground committee with whom the SCP worked, the steering group met to plan the public meeting and used the planning session as an opportunity to involve people who had shown interest when they had been petitioned. The worker's account of this process, which follows below, indicates her role in supporting individuals to strengthen the functioning of the group:

'Several of the people we had called on during our Sunday morning canvas attended that meeting (of the steering group), one of whom was shortly to be the first chairman. But a number of the people whom I had hoped would attend did not. This precipitated the first of what were to become frequent meetings between myself and the curate to discuss how we could ensure that the committee sustained itself. At the first meeting we were concerned about the pace of activities and this was a theme which recurred constantly. At this time we felt that the steering group might be doing everything so quickly that when the public meeting took place people would feel left behind. Later when the group had to go through the interminable waits for the council to reply to letters or to recruit a suitable worker, it was the feeling that nothing would ever happen that would threaten the group. At this point we decided that we should put some effort into extending the steering committee by talking with other people who had shown interest but had not attended any of the planning meetings. By this method and by small acts such as calling for people on the way to meetings I think we were able to encourage people who did not usually attend meetings.'

The steering group usually formulates the aims and objectives of the association, which might be part of a formal constitution, and which are presented for discussion and adoption at the first public meeting. Tension and discord may appear at this stage if the community worker or group members seeks to commit the group to what they believe are the most important political principles or problems confronting the group. Members may be seeking different things when they formulate a constitution including means to increase participation in the group. The steering committee of one tenants' association decided to concern itself with the poor maintenance services on the estate because individual complaints were largely ignored by the housing authority:

'There was a great deal of discussion [wrote the worker] about whether they should regard the impending rent rise as an issue which they should take up. Eventually it was agreed that they should not initially, as the tenants were divided as to whether it was justified or not. It was felt that it might prevent a strong association being formed if this issue was taken first.'

This period of discussion is often exhausting and depressing for group members. But it can provide many opportunities for an activist type of worker to influence the group's aims and objectives. He is influential if only because of his knowledge and experience of how other groups have coped with similar tasks.

The group should consider whether in the constitution the worker has membership and voting rights. If the worker does not expect to take executive responsibility in the group he must refuse invitations to do so without undermining the morale of the group or appearing unsupportive. In the early stages of their contact with the worker many groups have difficulty in understanding the roles that the worker finds suitable to take. At this stage of a group's development the worker should also be wary of other professionals taking on roles that might be harmful to the group. For instance, an SCP worker wrote about a meeting of a steering committee of a tenants' association:

'The vicar attended and thought he might have to take some chairing function, but after talking this over he took a back seat. This is one of the jobs a worker often has to do, preventing destructive action by one or another individual in the group.

In this instance, the issues were clear-cut since the individual was the local vicar and a worker would find it easy to justify speaking clearly about the inadvisability of him taking a substantial part in the tenants' meeting.'

Workers may find it difficult to raise such issues when the person is a tenant. Nevertheless, to do so may be essential for the viability of the group. It is usually more possible when the worker has warm informal relationships with individuals so that these problems can be talked about easily.

The Identification of Resource Decision-Makers

The worker can play an activist part with considerable impunity in helping groups to identify resource decision-makers but there is usually little need for this. The worker is not the only source of information available to identify decision-makers. Other groups can provide this information, especially where there is a common resource administrator like the local authority or the Greater London Council. The local newspapers and the secretaries of a project act in similar capacities. SCP had a store of knowledge of resource decision-makers in the form of a card index giving details of the persons and groups with whom the Project had been in contact.

The worker makes information available on who the decision-makers are and their range of powers. For instance, the worker helps a group working on slum clearance to learn about the clearance powers of the local authority; compulsory purchase orders; the procedures at public inquiries and rights of appeal; and the local authority's responsibility for rehousing tenants from a compulsorily purchased building.

The worker also assists groups to determine who influences resource decision-makers. If a group is negotiating with the planning officer for permission to open a playground on a derelict site they will want to know who the chairman of the planning committee is; the leader of the council and the local councillors; the local Members of Parliament and the political set-up in which they operate; and local press and television contacts known to be sympathetic to community action groups.

The worker helps residents identify the other groups in the borough or city who have concerns similar to theirs. This inter-group contact provides opportunities for groups to learn from and be encouraged by others' work. It broadens their horizons and objectives. When a playground committee was discussing whether it would provide a conventional or adventure playground an SCP worker arranged visits to playgrounds, slide shows and talks from experts on recreation. When the committee was recruiting its first full-time workers, the worker planned some discussions on playground work, led by various 'experts' in child care, delinquency and group work, who presented short papers and led discussions on the problems that arise in playground work. People found that discussing their own experiences with children in a generalised way seemed to make them more confident about their ability to select a worker.

While information-giving seems to be a fairly straightforward task, it is not distinct from policy-making. The kind of information given or withheld by the worker can determine the issues that a group takes up and the manner in which they go about their work.

Developing Skills and Confidence within a Group

This phase of interaction with neighbourhood groups demands more of the community worker's time, energy and skills than any other. It is the phase during which there seems most demand for the worker to be activist in his role, and the phase in which neutrality or non-directiveness seem to be most harmful.

Membership and executive responsibility in community groups demand a variety of skills that many people have to acquire for the first time. Many residents will have acquired these skills in other settings but need to modify them for effective use in neighbourhood groups. For instance, a tenants' chairman in north-west Southwark was sometimes criticised by members who thought he ran the association as if it were a trade union.

The tasks facing a group will include:

drawing up agendas;
promoting participation and task-sharing within the group;
writing letters and implementing group decisions;
maintaining contact with constituents through general meetings, leaflets and newsletters; and
coping with financial arrangements.

These may seem to be relatively straightforward tasks and many professionals may take them for granted. It may also be difficult to understand the extent to which groups in their early stages have to struggle to cope with means of negotiation that are culturally unfamiliar. The SCP worker with the playground committee, for instance, wrote of an early meeting of the group:

'The worker was already being put to other uses by the group. In a note to her following the meeting, the group secretary sends letters for typing, asks her to find out details of local trades councils and says: "Everything enclosed will need tarting up; grammar, spelling, etc. You will, I hope, do your best." At the next meeting, a letter from the Town Clerk, which ran to 500 words, was discussed. The letter said that he thought it would be more useful if the petition was discussed by representatives of the relevant committees rather than presented to the full council. It also asked when and at what times the committee could come and who would be coming. The committee spent some four and a half hours discussing the letter, and probably one and a half hours were spent in trying to decipher the officialese in which it was written. Eventually the committee decided to write back giving a date, stating a time which fitted in with the evening jobs of committee members and stating who would represent them. Not only did a letter come back giving an inconvenient time but when the delegation did arrive for the meeting one official said that she hoped there weren't going to be "too many of them". The worker was dispatched at past midnight to deliver the reply by hand to the Town Hall.'

This passage indicates the kinds of difficulties the group faced in negotiating by letter and deputation. These unfamiliar modes of negotiation may be seen, sometimes realistically, as instruments to frustrate the aims of groups. Delay, said Parkinson, is the deadliest form of denial, and so it must seem to many community groups in negotiating with local authorities. The worker writes of a meeting between the playground committee and the chairman of the Planning Committee:

'He was obviously surprised to be told very crossly by the committee that all they got were promises, not action, and that it was difficult to keep people hopeful with promises. They forcibly expressed one of the constant problems for local groups trying to obtain help, funds, land, information or service from local authorities – that of the crushing effect of delay. It is here that the local authority's power becomes only too apparent. The power to delay, to take the "necessary" time, to give no explanation as this occurs, can be one of the most damaging experiences for a group and constantly underlines for them that they have little cutting edge with the bureaucracy.'

The amount of time the worker spends on tasks like writing letters, minutes and funding applications varies with the experience and background of the individuals concerned. The playground committee, for instance, was aided by finding a lady who lived and worked locally and who could do shorthand and typing. She kept minutes, produced agendas and generally ensured that work agreed to was undertaken. Other residents with whom the SCP worked had their first experience with committee skills in these community groups. The worker not only aids in the development of these practical skills but also fosters relationships in the groups. SCP workers, especially new ones, were often given a variety of seemingly mundane tasks. These proved important in building a group's feelings of trust and confidence in the worker which broadened the range of roles open to him in other spheres of interaction such as in policy-making and negotiations with resource decision-makers.

We look below at the role of the community worker as he helps residents to share work, cope with finances and care for the group and its members.

1 *Sharing work.* It is important for the worker to promote the sharing of tasks and responsibilities within the group. This ensures that:

no person monopolises knowledge about the work of the group;
individuals are not over-burdened;
people acquire experience in the various committee offices;
individuals in non-executive roles contribute to the group's work.

The worker's role in this is illustrated in the following account:

'Mrs W, one of the secretaries, worked out the pattern of the meeting and rushed about the estate getting problems from all quarters. Everything from leaking pipes to truanting children came her way. She found it difficult to share the work with the other committee members but made such effective efforts to cope that the other committee members soon began to refer everything to her. This often seems to occur in the early stages of neighbourhood groups. To encourage a new group to share work in some way is a difficult task for a worker and I have often been unable to do this until the early "leader" had found it all too much and dropped out. Once this has happened groups have some experience of the necessity to share work and also the gap left by such a person makes a cut-up of the work vital.'

2 *Financial arrangements.* Coping with finance is a problem that faces many community groups, and Thompson has indicated that it was a problem that confronted early friendly societies.[1] Groups vary considerably in the extent to which they have financial affairs: a playground committee might have a budget of several thousand pounds a year whilst most tenants' associations deal in smaller sums that come from membership fees or donations for Christmas parties from local charities.

Groups often find it difficult to sustain people in the role of treasurer. Raising money has its enjoyable side and it provides groups with concrete evidence of success. But it creates anxiety. Many people are reluctant to take the treasurer's job thinking it will be complex, time-consuming, and lead to unpleasantness.

Besides being a worry and a source of work, finance may be a source of temptation and self-doubt. For instance, an SCP worker writing about a tenants' association said:

'Several committee members came to me in the week to say that they were unhappy at the way in which Fred had conducted the raffle. There certainly did seem to be a large discrepancy between tickets sold and money returned, and Fred could not produce any receipts for the money spent on prizes. My suggestion was that they ask him about the raffle before the meeting, but in the event it was raised at the meeting itself and Fred resigned on the spot in a huff. No one was then prepared to take on the job of treasurer and most of the committee said they couldn't trust themselves with the money. "We know we'd use it when we ran short in the week." '

[1] Edward Thompson, *The Making of the English Working Class* (Gollancz, London 1963), p. 419.

It is tempting for a group in this kind of situation to look to the professional to administer its monies. Handling large sums of money, keeping accounts, taking and giving receipts for cash transactions, opening bank accounts, and presenting a treasurer's report were tasks that often made people feel inadequate, and the SCP workers often found it necessary to help a group with these difficulties. At one stage in the life of a group an SCP worker became its treasurer. This worker wrote:

'Everyone refused to take the post and no amount of encouragement or cajoling on my part could change people's minds. No one would trust themselves, and most seemed overawed by the cheque for £70 which the BBC was sending to the group in the next few days. The trouble with Fred's raffle was only the culmination of several weeks' anxiety in the group about money matters, an anxiety which did not help the group to focus on its primary tasks. After much discussion with my colleagues in the Project, I reluctantly accepted the post in order to help the group forward. I accepted, on the condition that I was co-treasurer with one of the tenants, and one woman volunteered immediately. I also explained to the group how accepting the post might change the role I played in relation to the group's business, and that it might prejudice the good relationships that had developed in the past. I said, for example, that if I was chasing the editor for newsletter subscriptions in my role as treasurer, this might inhibit the way in which he would relate to me in my role as community worker. This is, in fact, what happened. A conflict developed over what to do with the money from a well-wisher. The argument went on for several weeks and relations were very strained between myself and some of the officers of the association who were clearly resentful that my role as treasurer gave me a position of control in group affairs which a community worker would not normally command.'

The appropriateness of a worker taking on an executive role in a group will depend on a number of factors which the worker must assess. In the example we have given, the worker decided:

that anxiety about finance was crippling the group at an important stage of negotiations with the local authority;
that he would, by becoming treasurer, encourage a tenant to

come forward as co-treasurer who would acquire skill and confidence in the treasurer role;

3 *Caring for the group.* The worker helps groups in the following ways: to cope with crisis and setbacks in their work; to recruit new members and ensure that officers 'train' their replacements; to attend meetings and implement group decisions; and to support individuals in the domestic and work problems that may affect their contribution to the group. This section confirms the need for consciously selected interventionist behaviour on the part of the workers, as he chooses the degree of activism or neutrality of his role according to the needs of the group and the problems that it confronts.

The worker assists the group establish means to recognise and deal with problems that arise within the committee. Part of the worker's job is to articulate the concerns that individuals have about the committee's functioning and to help individuals deal with their fears and anxieties. In the SCP we found that group members were frequently concerned with the following problems:

the political affiliations of committee members. For example, members felt that the politics of the local communist candidate who helped the playground committee 'might put other people off';

the political attitudes and motivations of the community workers; the slow pace of community work. Committee members became despondent if they were unable to give friends and neighbours news of progress. Complaints about lack of progress are also a way of expressing criticism of individuals on the committee;

loss of committee members. This was a common problem to community groups. People left because of disagreements, rehousing outside the area, ill-health, domestic worries and loss of interest; the SCP workers kept the question of *renewal* and *recruitment* on the agenda of groups. The problem of membership loss varied from group to group. One tenants' association, for instance, working in a block for homeless families accepted the inevitable loss of committee members as families were rehoused into the normal housing stock. At the same time, resignations and votes of no confidence occurred frequently in this group

as a means of dealing with problems that would be resolved less dramatically in other groups, though offending members were usually recruited back. In most groups, resignations breed doubt about the group;
differences in attitudes to advice; this is one of the factors that leads to disagreement within and, sometimes, between committees. Advice may be seen as a directive or a criticism if a person's life experience has not provided chances for making decisions by weighing alternatives. This was noticeable in a playground committee comprised of a number of people with different skills and backgrounds. Thus, the worker writes:

'When one committee member says the books should be kept in one form, the treasurer might feel that this was a directive and that to ignore it put her in direct conflict with the advice giver. Conversely, the playground worker who had had a traditional arts education took what he viewed as advice as comment, to be weighed with other views. This sometimes made committee officers feel that he was unwilling to do what the committee wanted. On many occasions the worker has been asked by committee members to work out what they wish to say at the next meeting, particularly when "advice" has been given which that committee member does not wish to follow. Sometimes the playground workers have also made use of the worker to discuss how to present their views in a situation where there are differing opinions concerning their work. Some committee members have found it took time to find a workable role as employer, particularly where they have been used to authoritarian employers themselves, but also where they have over-identified with the playground workers as the underdog.'

The personal matters that concern committee members often impinge on meetings and seem an essential part of them. Difficulties about getting jobs and houses, the court cases people get involved in, personal successes in getting new jobs, bargains or winning at bingo, social events, weddings, parties, and funerals are all mentioned or discussed, sometimes during a meeting but more usually in the time preceding the meeting or after the meeting closes. At such times the worker can give information about services or comment on the issues raised. For example, a committee member told the worker how he went to his son's Open Day at a local primary school and asked his son's teacher if there was any way he could help his son educationally. The teacher replied that he should keep out of things that weren't his concern. The worker thought that the man was seeking some reassurance that the teacher behaved offensively and the worker expressed disapproval of the teacher's behaviour. However, the worker may not always be sure about the appropriate way to react to overtures for personal help and reassurance. It is necessary that the worker be prepared to offer sympathy and attentiveness which is, frequently, the thing that people most want and need.

The personal behaviour of members may impinge on the work of a group. For instance, members of the playground committee frequently approached the worker to discuss what might be done about something another member was doing. One member often giggled at meetings and other ladies felt anxious about it. The worker discussed with them why she might giggle and how they might prevent this. Other such discussions concerned committee members' drinking, love affairs, language, bossiness, unreliability, tetchiness, pettiness, failings as a chairman, alleged misuse of money, poor record keeping, unfairness, dishonesty, and so forth. Almost every committee member was at some time criticised by others for their failings. The worker's function was neither to defend the member being criticised nor join in the abuse. Rather, he helped members to sort out their observations and to assess the situation from the point of view of the objectives of the group. In his work with members and with the individuals being attacked, his interest was in helping the individual to act in ways that would be useful to the individual and to the group. Of course, this may not be an easy or comfortable task because the 'best interests' of a particular group are not always consonant with the 'best interests' of a particular individual.

Not only does the worker provide support to individuals, but the committee can do much in caring for its members. When the treasurer of a committee was admitted to a mental hospital, the members sympathised with her husband and offered to care for her child. The worker was asked to visit her because it was not possible for committee members to get to the hospital in Surrey. In this situation the members and the worker were part of the internal support resources of the neighbourhood.

In helping a group to sustain itself it is often necessary for the worker to intervene deliberately to support the group and individual members by providing advice and encouragement. In interacting with neighbourhood groups the community worker has a responsibility to assist the group actively in caring for its organisation and morale.

Negotiations with Resource Decision-Makers

Policy discussions in neighbourhood groups are, like those of the local authority, concerned primarily with the acquisition and use of resources over which the group has influence. The resources are used to promote the aims of the group although some resources such as a project's telephone may be used for the personal purposes of group members. We have noted that many groups worry about group resources being diverted by members who are short of money. But resources might be used in this way by policy of the group. One tenants' association, for instance, made loans to families who ran short before pay day. Here, though, we will be concerned only with resources that local groups can use in negotiations with resource decision-makers. Besides the individual and collective skills and strengths of the group an important resource is the community worker himself. Thus, it is necessary to understand the relations between a group and a worker in the formulation and implementation of policy and strategy.

It is useful to distinguish between the primary aims and objectives of a group and the secondary areas of concern that it develops from an increasing awareness of the needs of its constituents. Most of the tenants' associations, for instance, with whom the SCP worked aimed to clear slum blocks and to achieve adequate rehousing of tenants; the playground committee sought to open and manage a playground; the group concerned with area redevelopment sought to oppose undesirable aspects of the riverside development. The worker contributed little to policy-making at this level: residents may have formulated these goals before approaching the SCP for help. But the worker's role may be crucial in defining and extending these fundamental ambitions. For instance, the tenants' association of the homeless families block was initially concerned with cosmetic improvements in their deteriorating environment. Partly as a result of contact with SCP workers and partly from contact with other tenants' associations in the area, this association developed the goal of attaining closure of the block; eventually their goal became that of securing the closure of all Part III housing accommodation in the borough. This extension of policy objectives was gradual and, of course, Project workers and other professionals with whom the association worked made some contribution.

There are a number of factors that constrain or facilitate the worker's contribution to policy-making. These include:

the risks involved to himself and the group if he assumes a dominant role in decision-making;

his assessment of the group's reservoir of skills and confidence; his own identification with the group and the degree of inclusiveness in the group's operation; if a group promotes maximum involvement of members, and if the worker is regarded as a member, then the worker will be expected to contribute to group decisions like any other member;

the extent to which the group discusses tactics and negotiations at a project; if groups use a project to telephone and write letters, it is likely that a worker's advice and comments will be sought when important letters and telephone calls have to be discussed and planned. If the group wishes to ignore the worker because they anticipate disagreeing with his views they can hold meetings elsewhere, such as in a member's flat or a pub. The worker can do likewise: there were, for instance, several occasions when SCP workers met with selected members of groups to discuss the work of the group. If other members learned about these meetings they were likely to be annoyed and upset.

An important factor in considering the worker's contribution to on-going discussion and implementation is that his contacts with members outside the group situation are probably as significant as his work at the group's regular meetings. Meetings are preceded and followed by discussion about agenda items and the events of the meeting. This social interaction among group members, with or without the worker, is useful because some of it will be about group policy and strategy. Discussion might be about objectives or a variety of other subjects impinging on the work of the group. Points of view put forward in these social contexts by a worker might be subsequently taken up by a member and adopted by the group at its regular meeting. The worker can use these social occasions deliberately to raise points that he would like to have taken up by the group; or the worker's opinions might emerge as a result of spontaneous discussion with members. These kinds of discussions help to build relations of trust and confidence among group members and the community worker. The worker is tested on a variety of issues: his political ideology and commitments; his reaction to neighbourhood activities like petty crime and his connection with professionals in the local authority about whom there might be both interest and mistrust. If the worker is accepted on such issues this will increase his opportunities for other successful interaction with the group. The complexity of the field situation makes any one conventional role designation seem nonsensical. The worker may be non-directive at a meeting where policy or strategy are discussed but he may have considerable influence on the outcome of the discussion because of his contribution to informal pre-meeting discussions. Community workers avoid being labelled as manipulative by being non-directive; it is possible only to clarify and never suggest, never to become a member of an organisation but to go only when invited, and to speak only when asked. But this does not mean that the worker does not considerably affect the situation.

The passive, inactive role might be eschewed for more practical reasons. Work with extremely deprived groups requires the worker to identify and share more fully in the group's operation than might be appropriate with other groups. Because the worker is 'unlike' the members because of residence, age, experience and education he may find that he is used by many people for trying out ideas. The worker may be unsure about how to be helpful without reinforcing feelings of inadequacy that may underlie the tendency of members to attribute excessive ability to the worker to solve problems.

The worker must respond flexibly and sensitively to each situation. There are times when a high degree of involvement with the worker may be dysfunctional; at other times the worker's intensive involvement may be necessary in order to help the group do its work. What the worker contributes of his own ideas and energy should be determined in part by the degree to which he is identified with the needs of the group. Moreover, the worker should share as much of himself, as a person and as a worker, as the group members offer him. For instance, one worker entering the SCP at its halfway stage wrote:

'I found that I had to establish good personal relationships and rapport with individual members before it was ever possible to make myself professionally relevant. The first few months were significant for the number of occasions in which some people invited me to tea to discuss their family and mine and to swap family photographs; others, especially some of the men, took me round the pubs; and others invited me to parties on Friday nights at their flats. There was a great deal of curiosity about my wife and child, about my background, my attitude and views on life.'

The need for this kind of sharing and identification varies inversely with the extent to which local people have grasped the meaning of community work as a helping profession. When the professional role of the worker is understood, the need for personal relations and understanding are of less importance. In the SCP, strong friendships developed between the workers and many of the members of groups, relationships that were important in helping to push forward the work of the groups. The point remains, nevertheless, that such relationships may be a source of covert influence for the worker.

The community worker is often used by neighbourhood groups as an instrument of negotiation. This can be illustrated by reviewing an SCP team discussion of homeless family tenants' association which appeared to be on the verge of success in closing and clearing the block. One Project worker argued that the council should be pushed to a decision by the Project. The Project, she argued, could advance the work of the group by taking a public stand against the conditions and stigma of homeless family housing in the borough. Other workers resisted using the Project in this way, arguing that if the tactic was successful the morale of the tenants' association would be undermined by confirming that, in the end, local groups have no cutting edge with bureaucracies and that decisions are effectively secured by dialogue between middle-class professionals.

The Project did not make a public stand on this or any other issue of the kind, but on a number of occasions the skills of individual workers were exploited by the group in negotiations with the local authority. We describe two types of role for the worker in these kinds of negotiations.

1   The high profile role – the worker might be given a task to achieve as part of the negotiating machinery of the group. The SCP worker with the playground wrote:

'The delegation to the council was also planned in detail; it was agreed that the secretary should begin by saying why we wanted the site, the chairman to follow with some brilliant photographs he had taken of the useless concrete play space provided outside a new local block, and that the women could "chip in" as they saw fit. The delegation of eight people arrived at the Town Hall, and the chairman delegated the worker to "chat up" the vice-chairman of the Libraries and Amenities Committee. After the delegation, the secretary reported on the meeting and congratulated all who had taken part, bar the worker; he said that everyone had been willing to lobby the councillors but the worker had hung back and that in the future she should not be so shy about speaking to councillors.'

The worker may also exercise influence through his contacts with resource decision-makers in the local authority or in central government. The worker will often be in contact with these people on committees, at conferences and through the worker's links with other institutions.

2   The low profile role – the worker's mere presence at deputations and demonstrations will be encouraging and supportive to group members. An SCP worker, invited to accompany a tenants' committee to a meeting with members and officers of the local authority, was given no overt negotiating role. He was only asked 'to come along with us'. Afterwards, the worker realised that he had been invited for several reasons:

to support and encourage the group by his presence;
to mediate between the cultures of the articulate and inarticulate; that is, 'to help us make sense of the big words they always use', as one member of the group put it;
to take notes of the meeting, to help the committee prepare minutes which would later be sent to the council for their approval, and to make sure the council 'doesn't get away with anything';
to act 'as witness' to what the council would say: his status as a reputable professional would help the group to keep the council honest;
to clarify and analyse the content of the discussion with the group after the meeting.

The worker's account reveals that in the meeting both elected members and the council officers attempted to use the worker as their instrument of negotiation by a very hearty display of friendship. This kind of cordiality can, albeit unthinkingly, undermine the position of trust that the worker has built up with the group. There were many examples of this on the part of the local authority officers. For instance, a Project worker records:

'My role with the committee was also somewhat undermined by the Director's actions at the meeting. He was effusively friendly to me and as a result the tenants were convinced that I must know about the plans which he was so cagey about. I had to say that I knew nothing of them, but I think it took at least two weeks for them to believe this. On several occasions they have been very careful to check that I am not employed by the council and also have made clear in the minutes of meetings that the discussions at the committee shall not be passed on to the Welfare Department staff.'

It may be difficult for professionals in the local authority to understand the community worker's low-profile role. One SCP worker records that he was invited to a meeting between a tenants' committee and an assistant director of social service and a housing estate officer. The worker remained mostly silent and passive throughout the meeting. It became clear to him that his role was not understood by the assistant director who found it difficult to comprehend why a fellow professional was not playing a role commensurate with his presumed level of education, skills and articulateness. The worker was embarrassed because the assistant director persisted in addressing many of her comments to him throughout the meeting. The worker's only contribution to discussion was to reject forcefully the estate officer's threat to close the tenants' youth club because of health and fire risks. The assistant director rang up the Project a few days later to ask the worker's colleague 'to do something about that young Mr L', expecting that the worker would be disciplined.

The worker's role in these situations is defined by the wishes of the group; we have seen that the playground committee delegated to the worker an advocate role while tenants' association expected the worker to have a low profile. It was common for such meetings to be preceded by a planning session in which the worker and the members would discuss the purposes of the meeting, what the group expected to achieve, and what tactics it would use. This preparation was not always 'successful'; a worker with a tenants' association that was negotiating with a housing association that had bought the block for conversion improvement wrote:

'Most of the tenants attended the meeting with the Housing Manager and Secretary of the Association. Before the meeting I had given the secretary a great deal of information on the Housing Association and on the Greater London Council's way of dealing with removal expenses, which is the main bone of contention between the tenants and the Housing Association. The two officers of the Association were very articulate and skilled in dealing with the complaints and questions of the tenants and it was clear that an air of depression was settling on them. I was angry with the slick and facile things which the Housing Manager in particular was saying. I decided to intervene and attempted successfully to get the information which the Association needed and to dispose of the Housing Manager's evasions. This seemed to encourage the group, who laid in to the Housing Manager just as vehemently as I had done.'

Thus, during the process of a meeting, the worker made the decision to throw off the low-profile role expected of him by the group. The gains to the group outweighed the risks involved: the adoption of an active role might have been dysfunctional if the Housing Association had been able to dismiss the tenants' claims by stating that they had been put up to it 'by young agitators in that community project place'.

Conclusion

The worker's degree of neutrality and activism varies with the four phases of interaction with groups. The worker's active intervention is most problematic in the formulation of policy and selection of group strategies, whilst there seems to be greater need for the worker to take an active role in helping the group develop and nurture the form of organisation it chooses for itself. The important factors that bear upon the definition of the worker's role include:

the age and sex of the worker;
the amount of time he has worked with a group and the degree of his identification and commitment to neighbourhood problems;

the stage of development of the group, its ability to evaluate the contribution of a professional worker, and its confidence to accept or reject this input on merit;
whether the worker is resident in the neighbourhood and has a personal interest in the work of the group;
whether the worker has a locus or role other than that of community worker to the group, e.g. as its treasurer or secretary;
the extent to which the worker has succeeded in helping people understand his professional role in their relations with him;
the worker's personality and the way he relates to people.

In the SCP, residents frequently reverted to criteria of this last kind: 'I don't think I could go to him for advice'; 'I think he is going to put too many people's backs up'; 'I couldn't get on with him'; and 'He hasn't got the right background: I mean, how can he understand our way of life and get on with us?' These comments indicate the extent to which personal rapport is the factor that neighbourhood groups (and, for that matter, professionals and employing agencies) use to evaluate the community work skills of candidates or new workers in a project. Professional references are of limited help. Perhaps references from neighbourhood groups with whom someone has worked might be more useful. Academic achievements may be seen as having even less value.

As we have noted, strong bonds of friendship often develop between community workers and many residents who serve as officers in neighbourhood groups. Naturally, people move in and out of groups and these relationships are constantly changing, but they are instrumental in the work of the group. Many workers may feel uneasy about these relationships because they suggest that the worker exercises power and influence covertly. For instance, one worker who was at the SCP felt that the closeness of some of the workers to residents in neighbourhood groups was dysfunctional. It inhibited the ability of groups to absorb personnel changes in the Project; it smacked of traditional casework and tended to buttress individuals in roles in which they were no longer useful to their constituents. The problem, however, is one of balance. It requires, on the one hand, achieving the kind of identification with neighbourhood and personal problems that many neighbourhood people expect of workers and, on the other, minimising the dysfunctional consequences that might ensue from this sort of intimacy between professionals and service consumers.

Chapter 7

A COALITION: THE MATERIAL RESOURCES OF A COMMUNITY PROJECT

The notion of a coalition implies that each of the parties has skills and resources that it makes available to its partners. This exchange pushes forward the interests of the coalition and helps the partners to achieve their goals. In this chapter, we shall examine the range of material resources that a project brings to the coalition.

The most obvious resource of a project is the building from which the workers and groups operate. The SCP's first neighbourhood office was lost when the site was redeveloped by the property owner. From 1970 to 1972 the Project was located on a major through-way from the south of London to the City and the dockland working areas. The premises were flanked on one side by commercial warehouses and the local public library, and on the other by a betting shop, a hardware shop, an industrial designer, a Welsh chapel, and an undertaker. The other side of the busy road had been developed in a piecemeal fashion and comprised several derelict warehouses, a petrol station, some neighbourhood shops, and a nineteenth-century slum.

The internal layout and physical appearance of the office were helpful in establishing relationships between the Project and its users. A large display window carried posters and notices on a large variety of matters ranging from a local baby-sitting service to information about rent rebates and free legal aid. A small plaque on the door gave the Project's name. By intent, the Project avoided any announcements that might suggest associations with official agencies like 'the welfare' or the local authority. The grubby and unostentatious appearance of the premises harmonised with the other services in the terrace. The Project's appearance promised no magical cures for social ills but, rather, symbolised the dependence of the Project on the power, latent and manifest, in the local community.

The street door opened into a small front room where the Project secretaries worked. The rest of the ground floor comprised a large meeting room and a kitchen. On the first floor were four offices, one of them for students and the others for the three staff members. The neighbourhood groups used the large meeting room for committee meetings and made varying uses of the Project's facilities to carry on their work. The informal atmosphere and setting fostered the interaction of residents during the day. Members of the groups could sit around and chat to one another without having to account to anyone for their time and activities and for the use of the facilities. Most groups used the building as the territory on which to meet personnel from various departments with whom they were negotiating. Residents acquired strength and self-confidence from being able to negotiate with different departments on their home ground at the Project, with files and documents available. This was a special convenience for members who might not have the time or the courage to venture southwards to the Town Hall. Local groups are easily intimidated when confronted by local authority personnel in an elaborate and formal council chamber.

ACCESS TO THE PROJECT

The Project secretary gave each group a key to the building so that they could have access at all times. Access to a telephone was sometimes invaluable for obtaining help for individuals or families in distress. Giving keys to the Project facilities signified that the groups were trusted members of the coalition. For similar reasons some workers would sometimes turn up slightly late for evening meetings so that it was the group who welcomed the worker rather than vice versa. Access by the users to a project premises provides a useful and instructive model to other agencies, and also makes sense of any claim that general files and materials in a project are open for users to read and use; people need privacy to read material that others have written. And access to a project in the evenings and at weekends allows users to meet without the distractions of staff members (whom they might want to exclude from particular discussions) and without the diversions present during the working day.

Key holding by groups was important in other respects. With access to the SCP premises in the evenings and on weekends the building became part of the neighbourhood's internal-support resources. For instance, several people who lived in bad housing in north-west Southwark came to use the SCP as a refuge, seeking warmth, comfort and friendship. Others used the premises to sleep rough for a few nights, either to escape from marital problems or to implement an extra-marital relationship. Residents used the Project telephone for personal business, and were encouraged to do do so because there were few public coin boxes in the neighbourhood. On some occasions, when the SCP was closed (e.g. Christmas), families borrowed the fan heaters for use in their flats. Several residents used SCP workers to stand bail, as referees for jobs and hire purchase commitments, and to borrow small amounts of money in a temporary crisis. There were, of course, disadvantages to such open access to facilities, the most noteworthy being that money or property were more easily stolen from the building, and that the telephone was used to make long-distance calls. When this occurred the SCP team asked the groups themselves to raise the matter at committee meetings and point out to their members that these calls were a drain on Project resources and hence detrimental to the interest of groups.

THE ADMINISTRATIVE RESOURCES OF A PROJECT

There are a number of facilities that groups find essential for their work. Perhaps the most important are the telephone and a secretary who is available during the day to take telephone messages for group members. The telephone is a vital instrument in the work of the group since it is used for contact with all kinds of groups and individuals. Along with the telephone, groups rely on other pieces of equipment such as the duplicating machine, photo copier, typewriter and, of course, on the project secretary who types letters, gives information and welcomes callers. The typewriter and duplicator are invaluable for turning out news sheets, petitions, broadsheets, agendas, constitutions, minutes, and all the other written materials that help a group to function effectively and to keep in touch with its constituency.

These kinds of resources are the instruments that people in executive and managerial positions take for granted in their work. They are almost exclusively available to those who make decisions and they are less likely to be available to those who are affected by such decisions. Such resources are not easily found in neighbourhoods like north-west Southwark, and usually only in neighbourhood-based services like the school, church, settlement, college of further education, adult education institute, and the offices of voluntary and statutory agencies in the social services field. Neighbourhood users would have to complete with the agency itself for the use of these resources assuming that residents would see the service as one that would provide this kind of help and that the agency would consider using its resources to support neighbourhood groups. In north-west Southwark, several groups were embittered by the rebuff they experienced from agencies they had approached for the use of resources. One group depended on a local church for many of its resources and had to pay relatively heavy fees for use of rooms. The group's worker wrote the following about how ownership of resources creates the opportunity for control or influence in the affairs of the group:

'It was at this point, when the committee members were feeling a degree of success at being able to get the use of the church hall, that they began to show a degree of resentment towards the contribution made by the priests during the meeting. They felt that as they were paying for the hire of the hall, and the hire of the room for committee meetings, and the hire for the advice centre, it was up to them to decide who came to meetings and how the committee used the hall. They resented the fact that people came from the church who were not invited. The problem is that they have to be dependent on the church and its resources. They could never decide anything without either one of the priests being able to use his veto on any proposal they wanted to. Because of their attendance at every meeting of the committee, the committee will never be able to establish its own objectives and decide on its own course of action.'

Of course, the Southwark Community Project was in ownership of the resources that were used by local groups and, therefore, obtained a large measure of influence in the coalition. But it was not the ownership of resources that gave the workers their influence; nor did SCP's proprietorship act as a threat to the autonomy of local groups. The groups' capacity for decision-making and action were not constrained by any fear that Project resources would be withdrawn in the event of a disagreement over policy between staff and its users.

One attribute of the SCP that is important to consider was that its function was never entirely clear to neighbourhood groups or to service agencies. It is interesting to note the variety of names that local people gave to the SCP: 'The Social Security', 'The Social Services', 'The Southwark Process', 'The Project', 'The Southwark Communist Party' and 'The Community'. Many local people believed the Project was part of the local adventure play-ground whilst others thought that the Project was some kind of business venture. One worker was told: 'It's marvellous all you people doing this work in your spare time, but what do you do over there to make a living?' Comments like these reveal that the substantive reality of the Project was that given by its telephone, typewriter, and the sympathetic and helpful attitude of the people who were team members and local users. The reality of other local agencies in an area that have these kinds of resources is more firmly based; their role in servicing neighbourhood groups is limited by their service functions and by the stereotypes and prejudices that have come to be associated with them. The near anonymity of SCP's auspices and the lack of clear definition of agency func-tion allowed local people to choose freely the particular resources of the Project that they wished to use.

Chapter 8

WORKING WITH SERVICE AGENCIES

We have indicated that one person in the Southwark Community Project was given primary responsibility for working with service agencies. It is important to note, however, that other workers who were primarily concerned with neighbourhood groups also interacted with agency staff in the borough; and that the SCP service worker, and others like students who operated with services, also had some measure of interaction with neighbourhood groups.

The SCP service worker, who had had twenty years' experience in the social services field, was located in the Project's neighbourhood premises. Not only was the SCP an 'outside' agency but the worker was to attempt her task from outside the formal structure of service provision. She was to co-operate with services whilst not being part of them, and to work with them in respect of the variety of service delivery problems and community needs described in Chapter 2. The Project's resources in this task were limited. It had little in the way of power, or authority or inducements; it had only the time, energy and ideas of its staff. Many voluntary agencies valued its autonomy and independence of local authority finance.

It was an early assumption by Project staff that collaboration and discussion would culminate in effective problem-solving. It was assumed that local social service agencies had the capacity and the will to divert resources and to adapt to changing needs, once agreement had been reached on the nature of the problem. Given limited resources, and the complexity of the service operation in Southwark, Project workers came to realise that the achievement of change in the services would have to be fought for. It was not viable to adopt the role of the passive consultant who sat back and waited for agency staff to come forward. The reality that emerged for the worker was like being a social vagrant, renewing contact by attending innumerable meetings, by making soundings in informal and formal ways, constantly looking for opportunities to develop working relationships with relevant service personnel. It became necessary for the Project worker to be visible and accessible in many settings, and to all levels of staff in the social services.

During its first months the SCP team initiated contact with senior officials in the borough in order to gain general support for the Project. The workers collected the views of different people about needs and problems and defined some areas where more detailed studies might be appropriate.

The team explored four geographic areas in different parts of the borough. Summary histories of these localities and land use maps were prepared which provided a description of the area, its facilities and open spaces, the density and characteristics of its population, housing conditions and the planning intentions for the area. Groups of social workers, health visitors and other personnel in the voluntary and statutory services were visited, including clergymen, school teachers, probation officers and settlement workers. Contact was made with residents through tenants' associations, playgroups and informal organisations. Data gathered from these sources were put together in 'area studies' which became working papers for team decision-making. These explorations provided an opportunity to get to know agency staff and to make an initial assessment of the services, their community relevance and the attitudes of staff towards the areas they served. Maps were also prepared which illustrated the variety of geographical administrative units used by services, few of which had co-terminous boundaries. These maps and area studies became information sources and visual aids to service staff, few of whom had time or responsibility to undertake locality studies.

Seeking Allies

Information gathered as a way of learning about an area and the services that operated in it was also useful in locating potential allies in agencies who had interests in common with Project staff. Discovering potential allies was considered important because of the assumption that any work undertaken for an agency would be developed in collaboration with individuals in that agency. Such collaboration was also necessary because of the time-limited nature of the Project.

The SCP workers initially found most support amongst some

chief officers and some field workers. There was less interest at
the middle-management level although some middle-management
workers did pay lip service to the importance of community work
as far as it was understood. In the early stages of the Project's involvement with services, a number of suggestions for collaborative
work came from field workers who were aware of the problems
of their agency and its users. An interesting example of this is
provided by a senior child care officer who helped to initiate the
Multi-Service Group on the Rockingham Estate.

Joining Efforts with Other Agencies
The Project workers found that their interests often coincided with
those of some service staff and, in particular, with those of the
planning department. This department proved to be an open one
and was an accessible source of information. The Project was
helped by the department's inter-disciplinary team of sociologists,
social geographers and planners. Several members of this department wished to work with the Project to develop the collection of
social data, and they were already preparing information that
would be relevant to the social services. Some staff in this department envisaged that the SCP might facilitate their aim of widening
the department's role in social planning within the borough.

Open Intervention
At the conclusion of the exploratory work, a letter was written to
everyone that the Project team had seen. It thanked them for their
help and told them of the decision to work in north-west Southwark. The letter also restated the community work objectives of
the team and outlined the responsibilities of its individual workers.
Recipients of the letter were encouraged to respond and to contact
the Project workers if there were any way in which they felt the
Project could be of help. The letter was sent to staff at various levels
of organisation because people were not necessarily informed of
correspondence coming in at the senior level. It was also distributed
to people in a large number of voluntary groups and services.

THE DEVELOPMENT OF WORK WITH SERVICES

The effectiveness of the SCP as a resource to service agencies depended on three variables: the behaviour of the worker assigned to
service development; whether agencies thought that they were

more likely to benefit than to lose through collaboration with the SCP; and the attempts of the SCP in maintaining its credibility with service agencies. We shall examine each of these.

The Worker

The behaviour of the community worker is of particular interest when the worker must operate outside the formal service structure. The worker has no entry to agency discussions, except by invitation. The worker cannot contribute to agency decision-making, except by invitation or perhaps through finding a 'spokesman' for her views amongst the agency staff. The worker has to be conscientious in taking up and creating opportunities to co-operate with service personnel in a number of formal and informal situations. The SCP worker, for instance, had to be ready to accept basic servicing tasks like convening meetings, preparing minutes and distributing agendas. She undertook any job that might offer opportunities for influencing the thinking and work of agencies. She endeavoured to influence staff through her enthusiasm, energy, charisma and dedication to the interests of the neighbourhood and to the development of appropriate services. The SCP worker also needed to be equipped with knowledge and information that agency staff would find useful; knowledge, for instance, about contemporary developments in methods, research and training in the social services, as well as information about the area.

The Service Agencies

A major task of the community worker is to identify for staff in services the likely benefits to them and their clients of collaboration with a community work project. The SCP was a small operation under voluntary auspices; as such, it stood the risk of either being co-opted by the major power forces in Southwark or of being ignored by them. The Project worker had to cope with this situation by establishing not just trust but an understanding of the reciprocity of interests to be served by agencies collaborating with the Project workers. It was not sufficient for the Project to assume that its definition of its purposes would adequately convey the ways in which agencies would benefit. Indeed, some Project definitions ('helping services to improve their community relevance') might have alienated officers and elected members. Because of this, it was necessary for the Project to develop specific pieces of work to demonstrate its value to service agencies. In this respect, the analysis and report on homeless families was a facilitating piece of early work.

Maintaining Credibility

It was a major task of the SCP service worker to maintain the credibility of the SCP as a resource relevant to the needs of agencies. There were many factors that militated against SCP remaining credible. These included:

the effects of neighbourhood work – the work of the Project with neighbourhood groups strained against the efforts of the Project to work with local authority agencies, some of whom were in conflict with neighbourhood groups or feared their 'interference' in service matters. For instance, when the team moved into a neighbourhood base, its ability to collect information from the welfare department and to influence its day-to-day workings was reduced;

staff resources – the time, energies and ideas of a small Project team were extremely limited given the size and complexity of the service operation in Southwark;

agency changes – the Project worked at a time when the social services were embroiled in the problems of reorganisation as they anticipated and implemented the Local Authority Social Services Act 1970;

lack of understanding of community action – the local authority's lack of experience and sophistication in the area of community action often led it to attribute neighbourhood activities that it found embarrassing or difficult to resolve to 'the hidden hand of the Project';

Project structure – the confusing nature of the Project's organisation, which was collegiate rather than hierarchical. No one person was 'in charge'; the local authority may have been deterred from collaborating because they felt that no one was responsible for the Project and the activities of its workers. The informality of relationships with local residents and their activities in the Project office (for example, answering telephones) may have compounded the reluctance of local authority staff to collaborate.

It was important that the Project's credibility be maintained and improved upon in order to influence senior and middle management in the services, and to secure work from them. The intentions and the integrity of the Project was not an issue in its early period; indeed, a good start was made with the enthusiasm, support, good-will and patronage of some of the chief officers and councillors with whom the initial negotiations for establishing the Project in Southwark had taken place. As time went on and the Project became more involved with neighbourhood groups, access to decision-makers and influencing policy decisions had to be struggled for. 'Resistant' departments or staff members were kept on the Project circulation list for documents and reports, and workers persisted in seeking their views and comments. In these ways, opportunities for dialogue were sometimes found. More coercive tactics were often used; for instance, by exploiting rivalries between departments or by approaching senior officers, councillors and local Members of Parliament.

Exploiting rivalries that existed between agencies was a tactic that helped to maintain the Project's influence. These tensions and rivalries sometimes facilitated work with specific services. For example, a department was less likely to refuse the opportunity to present its views if it saw that other services were taking the lead. But it was never sufficient merely to exploit such rivalries. It was the task of the worker to develop co-operative planning among services and this was dependent upon mutual interests being served, knowledge of respective functions and roles and a genuine concern for improvements in service provision.

Conflict between agencies and tensions between agencies and the SCP provided growth points. An agency might agree to collaborate because it sought to protect its own interests, to safeguard its own power position by not wanting to appear resistant. Yet this might provide the outside community worker with a way in and lead to services becoming more aware of other's points of view. Another example is the number of occasions when senior officers from the departments of the town clerk, social service and housing telephoned with an urgent point for complaint or discussion; they would ask the Project's service worker 'to control' the neighbourhood workers, the students and even the community groups themselves. It was often possible to use the complaint or discussion to illustrate what the Project work was about or to explain why it was not possible to deal with their complaint in the way they wished. This also helped to illustrate that team members were not in direct control of actions being taken by neighbourhood organisations.

AN EXAMPLE: THE ROCKINGHAM ESTATE MULTI-SERVICE GROUP

The Rockingham Estate Multi-Service Group was an inter-disciplinary group of fieldworkers to whose formation and functioning the SCP service worker contributed. It started in 1969 and continued to meet after the withdrawal of the SCP. It served to link personnel in a wide range of social services, all of which had as part of their catchment area the Rockingham Estate, a large inter-war GLC development. The Group also included representatives from the local community.

From the point of view of the SCP, there were three purposes in initiating and developing the Multi-Service Group:

to promote better co-ordination between the helping services;
to assist services to become more able to meet the needs of the community by establishing a dialogue among staff, and between staff and residents. It was hoped that this sharing would lead to a wider examination of the nature of the problems encountered by both agencies and consumers;
to illustrate the inter-dependence of services and to indicate the common bases from which they operated in their responsibilities to one particular locality.

We shall examine some of the major tasks carried out by the Project service worker in her contribution to three areas in the development of the Multi-Service Group.

1 Initiation

As part of the task of identifying areas of need within north-west Southwark, the Project worker had asked a senior child care officer to analyse the children's department's cases on a geographical basis within the Project patch. This analysis indicated that most officers were visiting the Rockingham Estate. The Project worker then suggested that the officers should visit their clients on the estate to discover what residents saw as the advantages and disadvantages of living there.

As a result of the analyses of caseloads and data on residents' views, the senior child care officer (SCCO) decided with her group to call a meeting of all staff engaged in services to that estate. She discussed this with the Project worker and together they prepared a list of all relevant people who worked on the estate. This list contained fifty-six names. The next task was to consider who might most effectively convene the meeting, and what would be the most helpful way (in terms of encouraging attendance) of describing its purpose. The selection of a convenor who could secure collaboration from others was a crucial judgement. It needed to be someone with a legitimate responsibility for social welfare and with an accepted and relevant position *vis-à-vis* the majority of services. It was also important that such a person did not appear to be using the role of convenor in order to attract more power to themselves or their agency.

It was decided that the SCCO would be the most effective convenor since the children's department had a statutory duty to prevent the need for reception into care and the court appearances of children. Here was a valid reason for bringing services together.

The next task of the Project worker and the SCCO was to draft a letter of invitation. This stressed the purpose of the meeting ('to enable us to get together and meet each other in person instead of by telephone, to gain knowledge of each other's work on the estate . . .') and its informal nature. It asked service staff to consider the possibility of further meetings; it also enclosed a list of those invited, partly because this ensured that people from some 'resistant' agencies would come if only to protect their own interests. The Project worker and the SCCO then prepared for the meeting by thinking through what might be usefully accomplished and how the SCCO might promote discussion. The Project worker records:

'The SCCO and I had a further discussion about the meeting and she discussed her notes. She said she was anxious that the meeting should·not appear to be a bid to take over power or prestige by the children's department. I reassured her that her valid reason for taking the initiative was because of the quantity of work that the estate was throwing up for her department. It seemed important that we should try to get this large body of people to agree that information could be collected from as many sources and participants as possible. By suggesting that they should go back to their users and to residents and ask them about life on the estate, they might overcome the feeling that they knew the whole picture from their specialist vision.'

Finally, the Project worker played a part after the meeting in picking up the responses of service staff to the meeting. Some staff telephoned to discuss what had happened and to seek help in thinking about contributions they could make in subsequent meetings. Whilst the service interest in the Group and in the problems of the estate began to grow, the Project began to explore the possibilities with the local rector of helping to build a residents' organisation on the estate.

Besides the tasks of working with SCCO to prepare for the meeting, the Project worker carried a 'safety net' role. This is revealed in some of the comments of the SCCO in her opening remarks. She referred to the part played by the Project in initiating the meeting:

'We might in a way *blame* Mrs X for this meeting, since it was a word that she said to us some weeks back that *forced* us to look at the actual area in which our clients live . . . this estate comes within part of the Southwark Community Project area and it is therefore an opportunity for us to spotlight during the five years of the Project's life what, if anything, we would like to happen here.' [Our emphasis.]

The statement reveals not just the SCCO's anxieties about convening the meeting but her desire to pass responsibility for it to the Project worker to safeguard the children's department should the meeting end in failure. It also protected the SCCO from being the primary target of any hostilities expressed by agency staff who doubted the usefulness of the meeting or who had been asked to come by their seniors. This was a particularly relevant role for the Project worker because most of the people present had very little experience of, or hope for, inter-service co-ordination beyond the traditional case conference.

2 *Group Maintenance*

The SCCO continued as convenor and was skilled in dealing with the delicate issues of inter-service relationships. The Project worker offered to take and distribute the minutes of the meeting and to assist any study groups established, hoping that the wide dissemination of minutes, documents and service information would encourage attention to local issues and problems from a wider audience. It was also a mechanism for encouraging attend-

ance and attracting recruits as service workers left their posts for
new appointments.

The Project worker and the SCCO tried to develop a structure
for the Group that was acceptable to as many of the members
as possible. There was no previous local experience among workers
of such an organisation against which they could measure the
Multi-Service Group. Thus, the worker helped to reassure and
encourage people who were uncertain or diffident about participation in a novel experience. The Project worker also endeavoured
to maintain as wide participation as possible in the Group's early
stages before people withdrew or left their jobs. Staff turnover and
changes in the representatives from residents' organisations often
raised problems for the Group about its cohesion and continuity.

The worker saw it as part of her job to facilitate relationships
among agency staff. She encouraged staff to discuss service problems in the Group and to share views with colleagues from other
departments. She supported workers who came to the Group without the support or enthusiasm of their agencies and she encouraged
them in their tasks of gathering and collating information about
their agency and its clients' needs for presentation to the Group.
The worker particularly helped those who were apprehensive about
the participation of residents whom they felt would inhibit a frank
exchange between services about the problems of the estate. The
Project worker was also able to resolve or mediate in inter-service
and inter-personal disputes and concerned herself with other kinds
of problems internal to the Group, such as bids for leadership.

The Project worker needed to recognise the diversity of motivations for people's continuing attendance at the Group. The reasons
people attended included:

gathering information about the estate and other services;
initiating contacts with other staff;
seeking support for an issue in which they were particularly
interested;
keeping a check on what was occurring in the Group;
effecting change in their own organisations which had previously
resisted a worker's attempts at innovation. For example, a medical social worker had struggled unsuccessfully to persuade her
hospital to provide more information about community care
services to elderly patients being discharged. She suggested a
letter from the Group to the hospital giving evidence of this

need which she then followed up in the hospital. After some
delays, the service was initiated;

gaining improvements in an agency's facilities. The local doctors
who attended saw that they stood to gain from the Group's
proposal for a multi-service centre;

focusing discussion on a wide range of issues of importance to
local people such as housing, rent collection, play facilities, the
poverty and problems of the elderly, the need for a community
hall, and communication problems between services and residents.

The proposal for a multi-service centre was a long-term, and
therefore safe, objective which everyone could support in principle.
It was an important ideal in itself but it also gave cohesion to the
Group and sustained its activities in times of depression or difficulties. The Project worker and others, however, saw it as their task
to draw attenton to the immediate, feasible and practical opportunities for service development and collaboration. These were, of
course, potentially more uncomfortable issues, as they reflected
diverse values and views about local matters and revealed the existing limitations in service provisions.

3 *Task Performance*
The Project worker contributed to sustaining interest and involvement in the work that the Group set for itself. This may be seen
in two areas:

the worker helped in the collection and collation of information
for various studies carried out by the Group. Her location outside the formal structure of service provision helped her collect
data from services on their provisions and clients. Services may
have been reluctant to share this with workers from other agencies within the authority;

the Group pursued its proposal for a multi-service centre from
July 1970 to January 1973 when a working party on the matter
was established by the chief executive, consisting of representatives from the Multi-Service Group and the Town Hall. The
Project worker not only sustained interest in the centre through
this period, but was also instrumental in drafting reports, plans
and letters, in organising deputations and delegations to the

local authority, and in helping to overcome chief officer opposition to the proposed centre.

This examination of the contribution made by the SCP service worker to the Multi-Service Group reveals how similar her task and roles appear to be to those described in previous chapters for the workers who operated with neighbourhood groups. The SCP service worker helped the child care group to identify a major problem area in its work and to formulate action about it. She then assisted in identifying those services who were likely participants in a collaborative exercise, and worked with others to define a structure and operating procedures for what became the Multi-Service Group. The SCP worker was further involved in helping the Group develop both in terms of its own survival and its capacity and willingness to carry through the tasks it set for itself. Finally, the SCP worker prepared and supported people in the Group in their negotiations with resource decision-makers (for instance, about the multi-service centre) and she herself was frequently used by the Group as an instrument of negotiation on delegations and at meetings.

THE ROLES OF THE WORKER

We can identify five major roles of the SCP service worker. They are as advocate, innovator/stimulator, adviser, informant, and co-ordinator. We shall discuss each of these in turn.

Advocate

There were four situations in which the SCP service worker assumed on advocacy or promotional role. She

1 persisted in pointing out to services the need to co-ordinate and plan their activities in order to improve what they offered to consumers;

2 encouraged agency staff to collect and use hard data in allocating resources, and in improving services;

3 advocated constantly that planning should not take place at the top of the political structures without consultation with field staff;

4 drew the attention of agency staff to the necessity and value of recognising the views of consumers and residents about service

provision. Whenever issues were being studied by agencies, the SCP worker pushed the agency to invite consumer participation in the studies, or to elicit consumer points of view.

The worker's skills in this role included being able to create opportunities for advocacy by, for instance, being seen as a valuable enough person to be invited to agency discussions, or interagency working parties. She had to resist being seen by agencies as a 'community spokesman'. Agency staff would often ask 'What do you think the local community feels about this problem?' It was the task of the SCP worker to suggest ways in which the agency could directly sound out local opinion. The worker also helped local people and agency staff to advocate for themselves in regard to service development. A fundamental assumption of the worker was that she sought to make her advocacy role redundant as local residents and consumers gained access to decision-making in service provision. Such access was seen as a necessary goal, but it would not in itself ensure either better use of data or joint planning and action.

Innovator/Stimulator

The SCP staff member worked with agencies to develop new approaches to service provision. It was part of her work to encourage staff to be creative and innovative in responding to service-provision problems. She came to be used as a sounding board against which agency workers could test out ideas and suggestions. For example, some written guides to services (e.g. for the elderly and the young handicapped) were produced as an innovative response to meeting problems consumers faced in using the available services. Likewise, the secondment of an area team social worker to the SCP was an innovation achieved by the SCP service worker. Also, the SCP worker was instrumental in encouraging the opening of an advice service on the Rockingham Estate as well as in developing the notion of a multi-service centre.

The approach of the worker in this role was to involve agency staff in new strategies and proposals. It did not seem appropriate that the Project should prescribe 'what the area needed'. The worker realised that initiatives had to be formulated jointly with agency workers if they were to continue after the withdrawal of the Project. It was thought that the more agencies were engaged in the formulation of decisions about pieces of work to be undertaken by or with the Project, the more likely they were to be committed to the outcome or consequences of such work.

Because many agencies were sensitive about the involvement of an outside agency like the SCP in their internal affairs, the worker became skilful in communicating ideas to interested individuals in agencies who had the opportunity to present these ideas in intra-agency discussions.

Adviser

The SCP service worker provided advice and consultation to workers in voluntary and statutory agencies. She attempted to be accessible to service staff either by telephone calls or personal visits. Her advice, and that of other Project workers, was sought on a variety of issues ranging from the professional development of a particular worker to the improvement of an agency's services. The SCP worker also contributed to induction programmes for new service workers and to departmental conferences and professional meetings. Several agencies, particularly settlements, asked for the Project to help them develop their programmes.

The worker provided support to staff in services who were attempting to change the ways their agencies were working. It was useful for the SCP to identify and work with individuals who had an investment in and understanding of the community but who needed the resources and support of the Project in working for change.

The Project tried to encourage workers who wanted to achieve more of a 'neighbourhood orientation' in their work. Service workers who had operated with a clearly defined role in a neighbourhood found it difficult to operate with clients in an unstructured way and to move from their concern with the individual's difficulties to looking at the neighbourhood as a whole. The Project learned from many social workers that they found it difficult to enter a situation with little knowledge of what actions they would be expected to take and to engage in collective activities with residents, many of whom might be their clients. The Project team did find, however, that if agency workers were encouraged to draw together the information they individually possessed about a neighbourhood their view of that neighbourhood was often modified, and more attention given to the environmental and structural basis of residents' problems.

Informant

As the Project became established it was approached by individuals and groups for information. Providing information to service workers and residents was part of SCP's work. This included collecting and disseminating information on local needs, and the structures and functions of services.

As the Project's experience and store of information grew, many people sought its help in obtaining information on specific geographical areas·or issues of relevance to them. The kinds of people seeking this help included field workers from various departments, group leaders, student supervisors, planners and teachers. The Project encouraged these contacts as much as possible, particularly from those who were working in the locality.

A monthly 'information session' was started for workers and others in the locality who expressed an interest in SCP activities. Students and new workers were sometimes sent along to these sessions by seniors and supervisors. The SCP workers would give out material and offer the use of the files and maps for extractions. Invariably, after information sessions one or more persons attending would seek more detailed information on an aspect of the work that had been described. Formal requests were made by some individuals for collaborative work, for information, or for help with projects in which they were engaged. Sometimes the team had relevant information or could exchange views and ideas with them which they could use.

The Project worked with various staff groups in examining local issues. The collection of information by these groups on how services were operating became a preliminary task with which the Project workers helped. Information helped to clarify the nature of problems and challenged some of the myths and fantasies of service workers and residents about local needs and service provision. Facts and opinions were collected about needs and available services for special groups such as the young, the old, the handicapped and the homeless. Residents' perspectives were usually included in these reports, which were used as a way of pushing forward discussion, clarifying issues and gaining commitments to further work from agency personnel.

Co-ordinator

The SCP service worker sought, first, to bring agency staff together for discussions about needs and provisions; and, second, to bring agency staff and residents/consumers into joint discussions. We shall examine each of these in turn.

1 *Agency interaction.* The Project attempted to bring staff from different services together for discussions about their agencies' goals, functions and common problems; they also supported developments arising from such meetings that aimed at improvements of services or publicising issues. The Project worked in the following ways:

by encouraging the formation of and helping to maintain *ad hoc* inter-organsational groups concerned with specific issues or geographic areas (e.g. the Rockingham Multi-Service Group, the Young Handicapped Study Group, the Communication and Information Group). Efforts were made to ensure that these groups represented both statutory and voluntary agencies. Residents and users of services participated in most groups;

by contributing to inter-service working parties, pressure groups and committeees. These included the Standing Committee for Under-fives, the Standing Committee for the Handicapped and a Working Party on Play (these groups were part of the Southwark Council of Social Service). The Committee of the Social Workers' Lunch Club was another group with which the SCP team worked to create a forum for discussion and debate. During this period more radical groups emerged such as Case Con and a local Child Poverty Action Group.

Within such groups the nature of the problems and issues affecting the area were explored. Information about residents' needs and about service difficulties were collected, and suggestions as to how services could co-ordinate and improve their work often emerged.

2 *Agency–resident interaction.* We have already noted that in discussions about service provision the Project worker stressed the importance of obtaining the perspectives of consumers and residents. Generally, agencies ignored local resources such as tenants' associations and other neighbourhood organisations. The SCP had the mandate and the time to ensure that such groups were not ignored. The SCP worker attempted to help residents and users see the value of presenting their views to service agencies, and

to encourage agencies to recognise the pertinance of obtaining such views; and, in addition, the worker helped each to acquire confidence in their discussion with one another about local needs and service provision.

There was anxiety about interaction on both sides. This was illustrated when some representatives of neighbourhood groups met some of the area team staff of the social services department for the first time at the SCP office. Both expressed doubts about going ahead with this meeting; both were anxious to know who the other side saw as being in the chair. The event was a revealing one; both residents and social workers gained much information from this initial step. It led to further developments such as the establishment of a weekly advice service.

Another approach to the work was to strengthen user and consumer groups in respect of specific areas of service. It was possible to undertake studies from which information on the users of services could be extracted. It was also possible to contact members of particular groups (e.g. a group of young adult physically handicapped people, parents using a local playgroup) and obtain their views about their experience with services.

This chapter, then, has attempted to convey the phases of intervention of the SCP service worker, and the kind of roles, tasks and skills of her interaction with service agencies operating in north-west Southwark. In the next chapter, we make a tentative assessment of the Project's work with services and neighbourhood groups. In addition, we attempt to indicate some elements in the problematic nature of such an assessment.

Chapter 9

AN ASSESSMENT OF THE SOUTHWARK COMMUNITY PROJECT

The Southwark Community Project was not seen as a laboratory for testing different models and methods of community work intervention. The team did not try to experiment with different approaches of working with neighbourhood groups and service agencies. The decision to adopt a dual approach, for instance, represented only one of several models of community work. This model was not adopted for research purposes but because it seemed to offer the best prospects for achieving change. This is also true of many of the administrative decisions made by the Project. For instance, the purpose of the decision to give keys to neighbourhood groups was not to test the effect of this arrangement but to help the groups be more efficient in their work. We cannot evaluate what the effect would have been on the groups if the Project had decided not to give groups a key.

The stated field objectives of the Project as they were seen by the National Institute were:

to assist community groups to articulate their needs and objectives, and to take collective action in respect of them;
to assist organisations individually or in combination to develop their work appropriately to meet the needs of their clients;
to assist organisations to develop joint planning and collaboration to meet community needs more effectively.[1]

These objectives clearly assume that community work was to be the method of intervention. But they do not indicate how the strategies and tactics were to be evaluated. Indeed, decisions about these matters were left to the workers in the field and these decisions were always made on the basis of what would best develop the work with neighbourhood groups and service agencies.

It is important to note that all parties – Project staff, users,

[1] The SCP also had training objectives, e.g. the development of teaching materials, the provision of placements for students, etc.

service agencies – did not subscribe wholeheartedly to these objectives; some actors had other goals that existed alongside of the field objectives formulated by the National Institute. In assessing the work of the Project, one must consider the extent to which other interests in the borough viewed the Project as successful in the light of the objectives and expectations that they had for it. The total Project budget for five years was in the region of £62,000 and it might be asked: Was it well spent? In the following passage a ·Project worker raises some of the questions and doubts that many other community workers have felt:

'Since the funding for the Project largely came from large charitable trusts, we had to concern ourselves with the cost and effectiveness of our work. £62,000 could have funded a playground for ten years, a nursery for five years, an employment agency for fifteen years, five local residents as workers for seven years. The list is endless but the residents were never asked. Once again they were given what some charitable organisation thought they needed.'

The passage indicates the difficulties of comparing the cost effectiveness of various resources and of choosing among them. It also indicates difficulties of defining the agents of choice: thus, if there is £62,000 to spend in a neighbourhood, do the councillors, or service workers, or local professionals in the churches and schools, or tenants' association, make the choice; or should the money be used to advertise the options and hold a local referendum to decide among them? If so, how can we be certain that residents understand the meaning and potential value of the options; can we be sure that the phrase 'community work project' or 'adventure playgrounds' convey similar meanings to all parties? Would we allow residents to use the money for a network of bingo parlours; or could they decide to provide an employment agency or housing association that discriminated against immigrants? The uncertainty and doubt conveyed by the worker's words would have existed if the money had been spent on, for instance, a playground or a nursery; we then might question whether the money might have been better spent on helping the community to define its interests and to take collective action in respect of them. As far as northwest Southwark is concerned, it is important to note that there are now two playgrounds in the community; this indicates that the

£62,000 has been used to draw even more money and resources into the area.

There is, of course, no reality to these choices; we cannot ask 33,000 people to make them because the money is not available for these other uses and resources; and it is never available for the local community to spend as it wishes. In the case of north-west Southwark, the money was given to an outside body to spend because it had defined its interest in providing a community work project in a deprived London neighbourhood. Likewise, the neighbourhood groups in north-west Southwark that acquired funds from Urban Aid and other sources received them for purposes the value of which they had decided on behalf of the neighbourhood. There was no question of these groups, or the National Institute, being given x pounds 'to spend as the residents decide in north-west Southwark'. The money was to provide specific resources and the assumption was that decisions about that provision lay in the hands of a defined group of people, whether residents or outsiders, who successfully applied for funds.

It might be argued that the residents and groups have given some kind of answer to these questions in that they have established two operations (the North Southwark Community Development Group and Southwark North Action Groups) with essentially similar functions; they have shown considerable persistence in developing this work independently after the termination of the Project and despite enormous obstacles.

There are other questions to ask: Could the money given to a group have been used to provide a better playground, nursery, or whatever? Could the National Institute and the Project team have made better use of the £62,000 in meeting the objectives they had set themselves? Could the £62,000 have been better used if the objectives had been different?

There are many ways in which the SCP workers can now envisage the work of the Project being improved upon; but if there are some things that could have been done better, there are others that might have been done less well. The basis of the assessments in this chapter depends on the value and faith that the SCP workers had in the ways they interpreted and carried out their community work roles. Other community workers might have acted differently and may not attach value to the achievements of the Project and its users that we have noted. Some people may not have given as much emphasis to the development of organisational skills nor

seen the need or value of the flexible approach to work that underlines much of what was done. There is a wide diversity amongst
community workers of skills, commitment, values, methods, and
work philosophy and, therefore, much latitude for discussion and
disagreement over what constitutes effective community work
intervention.

Despite these dilemmas and the uncertainty of cost effectiveness
comparisons, there are a few questions we can ask that seem important:

> What would have been lost to the neighbourhood and the agen-
> cies working within it if the Project had not come into the
> neighbourhood?
> What would have been lost to the social services field and to
> training in community work if the Project had not been estab-
> lished?
> What were the Project's opportunity costs?

It is not wholly realistic to say that without the Project the
slums would not have been cleared or the playgrounds opened. It
can be assumed that at some point the local authority would have
cleared the slums and provided playspace and that at some point
local groups might have undertaken to prosecute the interests of
the neighbourhood. The crucial phrase is 'at some point', and we
suggest that had the Project not been in Southwark there would
have been delay in achieving the clearance of slums, the provision
of social amenities, and the formation of groups around neighbourhood issues. But there is, of course, a cost to delay, and the financial
and social cost of this delay to residents and the local authority
would be considerable.

The cost to the social services field is difficult to assess. By 1970,
the Project was only one element in the rapidly increasing commitment to community work intervention that had been expressed
by a wide range of local and central statutory and voluntary bodies.
From the National Institute's point of view, the community work
option for students might have been less satisfactory if the opportunity of field placements in the Project had not been available.
But the Project produced little teaching material and staff members
made only intermittent contributions to teaching at the Institute.
Certainly the Project produced experienced community work
practitioners with skill in teaching at a time when they were thin

on the ground. Some National Institute staff felt that there was insufficient commitment on the part of Project staff to teaching at the Institute and insufficient contact and exchange between the Institute and the Project. On the other hand, staff at the National Institute felt they had benefited from some of the documents produced by the Project and others in Southwark and that the Project had enabled several staff and students to understand the reservoir of ability, drive and intelligence to be found in deprived areas. The Project's work helped to convey a sense of what was possible if people operated collectively to achieve change, and many staff and students found the contribution of north-west Southwark residents to seminars a source of inspiration.

Finally, there may have been important opportunity costs of the Project's work in north-west Southwark:

1   There is a possibility that the Project may have pre-empted more radical protest, diverting people from protesting against the underlying structural causes of their poverty. There is, however, no evidence that this was an opportunity cost of the Project's intervention. It may be the case that residents active in community groups became more aware of the need for more fundamental protest as a consequence of their involvement in community action at the purely local level.

2   The Project was a time-limited intervention. We must ask, therefore, whether this inhibited similar activity by more permanently based neighbourhood institutions such as the Blackfriars Settlement. Even if this was a cost of the Project's intervention, we must weigh it against the work of Southwark North Action Groups in initiating a community work base as a locally-managed resource.

3   The Project's intervention could be counted as a cost if it had resulted in local service agencies rejecting their own responsibility for social intervention because of the presence of the Southwark Community Project. It would perhaps be a cost to the community if SCP's intervention had inhibited the social services department from making better, quicker and more permanent commitments to community work. Local authority departments are not generally renowned for the facility with which they embrace community work. It would have been an additional cost if the Project's presence had retarded the development of community work from

within the social services department of the London Borough of Southwark.

Opportunity costs of this kind must be weighed against the benefits to the neighbourhood that were a consequence of the work of the groups who used the Southwark Community Project. We attempt to delineate these benefits in the remainder of the chapter by looking at:

changes in the use, allocation and enhancement of neighbourhood resources;
changes and developments in individuals and groups;
changes in the work of service agencies, and in the attitudes of service personnel; and
the situation after the withdrawal of the Southwark Community Project.

1 CHANGES IN THE USE, ALLOCATION AND ENHANCEMENT OF NEIGHBOURHOOD RESOURCES

The Project was concerned with needs and objectives that were susceptible to change at a local level. There was no expectation, for example, that the Project's work could make any impact on the national structure of employment and income. The overall objective was also hedged with implicit qualifications. There was, for instance, no expectation that the Project would encourage people to engage in action that was violent or destructive of people and property. So the needs and objectives with which the Project was concerned were those susceptible to change via pressure and influence on resource decision-makers at the London and borough-wide level. Furthermore, it was expected that the means and methods of achieving these aims would fall within normal democratic practices of achieving change.

Housing

When the Project came into the area there was a large number of slum blocks of which the most infamous were Queens Buildings, Red Cross Way, Chaucer House, Goodwin Buildings and Guinness Buildings. There were, of course, slum blocks other than these which have in the course of the Project's existence been closed down and with which the Project had little contact. There were other blocks in the area with sub-standard accommodation with which the Project had no contact. In some of these landlords had attempted to improve facilities by extensive rehabilitation of buildings. The blocks with which the Project worked gave rise to tenants' associations which, to varying degrees, used the facilities and resources of the SCP. Queens Buildings, Goodwin Buildings, Red Cross Way and Chaucer House have all been demolished. Thus, structures of low neighbourhood value have been eliminated and replaced with facilities of greater value to the neighbourhood. The Queens Buildings site, for instance, has new housing and the site in Red Cross Way will have a new infants' and primary school.

The demolition of these slums means that the deployment of organisational support services to meet the pathology caused by sub-standard housing conditions is no longer necessary. The clearance of a slum leads to the reallocation of support services such as social workers, public health inspectors, probation officers, police, and fire brigade. The clearance of a slum means not only the reduction of pressure on local schools and lowering of numbers in classrooms but, more important, it means that new accommodation will help children to make better use of the school. On the other hand, the disappearance of hundreds of families away from this neighbourhood had the consequence of forcing several shops and services to close and this was detrimental to the population that remained in north-west Southwark. Also, the rehousing of people away from the area represents a drain of leadership from the community, though SCP workers always found that roles in groups were filled by people who had the required resources and skills.

The tenants' associations that were concerned largely with the improvement of maintenance and recreation facilities on estates also provide examples of success and achievement in their work.

Playground Provision

The two committees concerned with playground provision, the Rockingham Adventure Playground Association and the Mint Street Adventure Playground Association, were successful in achieving their aims of neighbourhood adventure playgrounds.

Redevelopment

The North Southwark Community Development Group was successful in: (1) promoting wider community understanding of redevelopment proposals; and (2) changing the local authority's redevelopment proposals for north-west Southwark.

Other Resources

Resources such as the local library and church gardens have been kept open as a result of initiatives from the Project and the neighbourhood.

Playgroups

A playgroup managed by parents for local children five to eight years old was successfully established on the Lawson Estate.

Advice Centres

A local advice session operates weekly on the Rockingham Estate, managed jointly by the Citizens' Advice Bureau, the tenants' association, and the church.

Multi-Service Centres

A community hall and multi-service centre is being constructed on the Rockingham Estate.

Social Service Surgery

A Monday night advice surgery is operated by the social services department.

Federation of Local Groups

A federation of local groups maintained a community work base in the area which employed its own community worker until April 1974.

This list provides examples of valuable additional resources in the neighbourhood; what remains problematic is the weight attributable to the coalition. How, for instance, do we weigh the contribution of the administrative resources made available to groups within the Project or the contribution that Project workers made to the development of organisational skills? We have already noted that these facilities were not readily accessible to groups elsewhere in the neighbourhood. Thus we can fairly say that these administrative facilities played an important part in achieving the goals of many groups.

2   CHANGES IN PEOPLE AND GROUPS

There was no explicit reference in the field objectives of the Project to the role of team members in meeting the organisational needs of community groups. But it was clearly assumed that the approach of Project workers would have a strong 'educative' element. There was no assumption about whether 'education' (the development of organisational skills) or the achievement of concrete objectives would have priority in particular developments. Some kind of inter-relation and balance was assumed but either might have priority in particular circumstances or at particular times.

The Project was not, however, concerned with adult education or community education as such; it was not a Project goal to im-prove levels of literacy, verbal skills, knowledge of civic affairs, and awareness of how government acquires and distributes resources. However, promoting knowledge may be the objective of a par-ticular group; the North Southwark Community Development Group, for instance, believed that community participation in the planning process must be preceded and accompanied by a pro-gramme of community education.

Although there was no explicit reference to community educa-tion in SCP's objectives, we have seen how a number of interests (including the workers, newspapers and more experienced groups) were engaged as part of their work in strengthening the knowledge base of neighbourhood groups. We described the need to maintain a flow of information to local groups on matters that affected their work; and, of course, groups strengthened this knowledge by learn-ing from their experiences. Their concern with knowledge was not an end in itself. The groups and Project workers attached impor-tance to this concern only to the extent that knowledge was rele-vant to developing the interests of the groups.

We can be reasonably certain about the acquisition of know-ledge. Groups did attain their objectives, which implies some success in acquiring certain kinds of knowledge. We are less cer-tain about other aspects of organisation skill development, namely, changes in the way people carried out tasks central to the work of groups. We outlined several of these tasks and skills in earlier chapters. The fact that groups continued to prosecute their aims in the face of many setbacks and were often successful is indicative of the achievement of confidence and competence in carrying out the kinds of tasks we described. Project staff did observe changes in people's abilities and self-confidence during the time they participated in the work of groups. These observations were often made in passing, as part of a general record of the work of the groups. There was no attempt to monitor the changes in the levels of individual competence and skill as an end in itself.

What weight should be given to the input of SCP staff in the process of individual change and development? The Project was the base around which many people cohered for varying purposes and periods of time. Skills and confidence were acquired from the interaction of these interests and from the experience of groups in prosecuting their aims with resource decision-makers. The workers in the Project were only one part of this interactive process. Of course, Project workers saw it as their responsibility to forward organisational skill development; and, of course, the workers were persistent in keeping this on their agendas. But the workers were only a part of a wider process of social interaction that affected the help they gave. But it is safe to say that people's skills and confidence developed from their involvement in these processes; the workers' contributions were significant because of the way in which they used their involvement to create opportunities for residents' growth. The worker's skill is, firstly, in the discipline he exercises in intervention; and, secondly, in the extent to which he can assess and judge his part in opportunities presented to develop the skills and confidence of others. He also assesses the ways in which residents exclude or open up opportunities for skill development. For instance, in an earlier chapter we mentioned how a worker dissuaded the local vicar from chairing a meeting so as not to restrict people's opportunity to participate in the work of the group.

Many neighbourhood residents' involvement in groups resulted in an extension of their knowledge and interests. Such involvement, because it took place within the coalition of Project workers and neighbourhood groups, often had the consequence of fostering interest and participation on a wide spectrum of neighbourhood issues. We will discuss this in two ways; first, by examining the effects of the coalition on individuals; and second, its effects on groups.

Individuals

Involvement in neighbourhood groups resulted in residents acquiring new interests and ambitions. At one level, individuals came to know more about housing procedures, rental and rate allowances, and supplementary benefits. This knowledge helped them and their neighbours. More significantly, this involvement led to upward social mobility; it is ironic that many local people aspired to the values and style of life of those with whom they had negotiated and Project workers with whom they collaborated. This struggle for self-advancement was not confined to Project users; two Project secretaries eventually took a social studies course and a teacher training course. Project field workers were given many opportunities to extend their skills and understanding as community workers and teachers.

Several residents applied for community work posts advertised within the borough; the secretary of one playground is considering attending a course for playgroup leaders at a local college; and the chairman of another playground wanted to work as a hospital visitor. An officer of a tenants' association, a welder by trade, took a job in a community development project. Project workers had some misgivings about these aspirations and achievements since they represented a loss to the local community. People were given the chance to move out of, rather than upwards with, their class and these aspirations and achievements are, one suspects, more the consequence of contact with professionals in the Project than of involvement in community action. Other workers in the neighbourhood shared the apprehensions of Project staff. One area team social worker told us:

'She and her colleagues were worried at what she called the unrepresentativeness of the few people currently pushing forward the work of the tenants' association. She also made the point that the kinds of skills which were being learnt by these few people were in effect removing them from the remainder of the tenants and aggravating their unrepresentativeness. The association of tenants with service people and other professionals on the Multi-Service Group served to enhance the isolation of these people from the remainder of the estate. She thought that the local tenants on the Multi-Service Group were assimilating the values of the service agencies about "clients and their problems".'

Continuing involvement in the work of the group and contact with other groups helped individuals to become progressively more confident about the kinds of tasks they took on. The boundary beyond which tasks and experiences were too formidable for them to contemplate was continually pushed back as people developed skills and confidence. There were, of course, instances of individuals becoming overwhelmed by the tasks confronting them despite the encouragement and support of the group and Project staff.

When we talk about Project team members working with groups we mean that team members related to committees elected by groups to conduct their business. Contact with the association's wider membership was usually confined to events like the Annual General Meeting, Christmas parties, outings, jumble sales, and day-to-day contacts in shops and pubs. The representative system meant that the worker usually operated with a committee of eight to twelve persons, though this number varied depending on the fortunes of the group in any particular period. If tasks were shared among committee members, the worker would normally interact with most of the committee. But no matter how well work was shared, most committees were run by a few individuals. This is not uncommon in conventional committee situations; many committees depend for their successful functioning on the drive of key members. Sometimes the committee's work places constraints on wider involvement in decision-making; the committee may have to respond to an urgent letter or telephone call or to a crisis affecting one of the members. In these situations, which seem to occur frequently in community groups, it may not be possible or judicious to postpone action in order to sound out all relevant individuals. Indeed, the flexibility of rules governing committee matters deliberately allows committee officers latitude to deal with situations that demand immediate action. With most of the groups using the Southwark Community Project, the worker had most contact with the officers of the groups.

Participation in the collectivity also varies from one event or experience to another; for instance, it is common for a large number of people to come to an Annual General Meeting, an outing, or a deputation or demonstration; but on the whole most constituents have their own domestic and work concerns and are willing to leave the running of group business to annually elected committees so long as they keep constituents informed of their work.

was very small, though it is difficult to assess how much of newly gained competence and ambition was passed on to others by the

The number of people who benefited from learning new skills

individuals concerned; and it is difficult to assess the impact these individuals had on others as a model for taking action on collective needs.[1] For instance, the success of a tenants' committee in closing a slum may have convinced some inactive members about the potential of collective action. It might be expected that many tenants will recall these experiences in the future when confronted in their new areas with the problems of deciding what to do about a local grievance. One can imagine that they would say to themselves: 'Well, why don't we do what old Mike and his committee did in the borough; it worked there so why not give it a go here?'

Many of the secretaries or chairmen of groups with whom SCP worked had had other experiences with collective action before they became involved in neighbourhood issues in Southwark. People with previous experiences and skills are likely to be among the first to emerge to fulfil key roles in group affairs. This happens naturally; the immediacy of the group's concerns, together with its uncertainty and diffidence, determines that those with some background of collective action are selected to prosecute the group's business. As the work develops, other group members with less experience acquire competence in handling aspects of the group's work. However, for many people, officer roles in community groups were often a recognition and enhancement of previous experience and not something new.

The Groups

A marked increase in the amount and kind of inter-group activity was noticeable in the last eighteen months of the Project. The North Southwark Community Development Group developed as a federation of groups opposed to speculative redevelopment and it included all the users of the Project; Southwark North Action Groups emerged as a federation of user groups determined to maintain a community work base after the withdrawal of the Southwark Community Project. The chairmen of many local tenants' associations met with the area team leader and some of her social workers. The meeting led to the initiation of a Monday night social service surgery at the Project offices; there was an exchange of ideas between the two playgrounds; and several tenants' associa-

[1] Jane Jacobs has given a good example of how community action skills are transmitted in a neighbourhood. See *The Death and Life of Great American Cities* (Penguin, London 1972), pp. 80–1.

tions worked together to plan a concert for old-age pensioners. This inter-group activity was made necessary by the needs of situations and it was made possible by the interests and abilities that had developed in several people. Hitherto, those active in community groups would not have been able to tackle issues that went beyond the interests of their particular group. Thus, the enhancement of skills and confidence by involvement in group affairs led to inter-group activity on wider issues.

Inter-group activity of this kind represents the achievement of certain standards of organisational skill development. But it posed problems for the groups such as several people becoming overburdened and over-committed. This occurred because groups diversified their interests in inter-group work but often failed to distribute new work and responsibilities amongst their members.

3   CHANGES IN LOCAL SERVICES

In this section we make some assessment of what was achieved in work with service agencies. The initial general objectives in respect of this aspect of work were:

to participate with statutory or voluntary organisations in thinking about how to develop their services in ways relevant to meeting community needs;
to contribute to the co-ordination and joint planning among services in order to meet these needs more effectively.

Any attempt in an assessment from the perspective of those involved is mainly speculative. It draws on reactions revealed by some who worked in the services. The assessment also includes information on some practical changes and development that occurred, but this does not indicate the precise nature or relative importance of a number of factors at work, one of which was the SCP. The assessment must be seen within the context of a particular period of time and take account of other forces that existed in that locality and that period. For some services, for example, it was a period of considerable change; the attempts of the Project to work with the social services took place at a time when these services were dealing with the problems of preparing for and implementing the legislation that followed the Seebohm report. Thus the timing of the Project's change efforts in respect of the social services was inauspicious to the extent that agencies were fully occupied with the large-scale issues of reorganisation.

We must also note other factors operating during the Project's attempt to work with services. The full-time involvement of one worker_with agencies was an extremely limited input, given the scale and complexity of services operating in Southwark. Second, the Project work with services was exploratory in the sense that there was little previous British experience in this area. Third, the worker was not based in an agency or attached to the local authority but chose to work 'from outside'; and we have already noted that the Project's involvement with neighbourhood groups constrained change efforts with services. Finally, the Project attempted to influence services at the area level rather than at senior levels in the management structure of agencies; Project efforts were largely geared to field rather than to policy changes.

We shall undertake the assessment by examing, first, the diverse activities of the worker responsible for work with service agencies; and, second, the specific outcome or products of this work.

Activities

The worker (and often her colleagues concerned with neighbourhood work) interacted with agency staff in a number of situations, and by telephone. Relationships were established in situations like the Social Workers' Lunch Club, study groups, inter-service committees and a variety of informal social settings. It is difficult to assess the contribution thus made by the SCP. There will presumably be some change effects associated with an SCP worker as a source of inspiration and advice. The Project was continually used by workers in services as a 'consultation point' on problems within the social services field. Workers from many 'helping' agencies approached SCP staff for discussion about relating their services to community work. We can presume that this contact helped at the least in the professional growth of service personnel, even though we can be less sure of changes implemented in, for instance, service provision and delivery. Workers may develop but they may not be able to effect change because of rigidities in the system of which they are a part.

One difficulty of this highly individualised impact upon the work of agency staff is that whilst many will have been guided and helped by SCP workers, others will have been alienated.

It is difficult, too, to assess the contribution that SCP workers made in official and *ad hoc* working groups concerned with the functioning of the social services. We may assume that one consequence of the workers' presence was that agency staff became more aware of the need and value of obtaining residents' views of services. Where SCP workers and others were successful in achieving user representation on working groups, an outcome may have been that service personnel came to recognise that north-west Southwark contained people of lively and determined abilities. To this extent, SCP work contributed in undermining the assumption of many workers that the community was pathologically homogeneous, without leadership or civic skills and responsibilities.

Finally, it is of interest that the activities of the SCP in north-west Southwark gave salience to an area hitherto neglected by both statutory and voluntary services. Both the neighbourhood and service agency aspects of the Project's work helped to enhance north-west Southwark as a focus for the attention of the local authority.

Outcomes

We are able to identify some specific outcomes from SCP work with service agencies that are, unlike those presumed above from the activities of the worker, relatively tangible. We look at each of these in turn.

1 *Reports and publications.* We refer here to documents which the SCP prepared, and to reports published in co-operation with other agencies in Southwark. In addition to published material, the Project made available data to service workers preparing internal or inter-departmental reports. Much time was spent with agency staff in collecting and disseminating information about the area. Apart from its value in the preparation of reports, the shared exercise of data gathering was useful because it:

illuminated different perspectives;
showed gaps and problems in the delivery of services;
made service workers aware of the views of residents and user groups; and
led to suggestions for new and different services to meet the wishes and needs of the locality.

In assessing this work of the Project we must note the time lag in the use of material by service agencies. For instance, the Project's report on homeless families was published in 1970 but it did not appear to be used by the acting chief welfare officer (whose predecessor had commissioned it) or raised by him with the council. But in March 1973, as the Project approached termination, a working party of councillors was convened to study homelessness in the borough, and the chief executive's department requested copies of the Project report for the councillors.

It is extremely difficult to assess the ways in which these reports affected attitudes and whether they were instrumental in achieving changes in service provisions or a better uptake of services by residents. There is some evidence but it is limited. We know, for instance, that hundreds of copies of the homelessness report were issued; that an early draft of the report was used by an officer in the welfare department to prepare a report for his committee; that the report advocated the redistribution of resources to give more housing units to those made homeless and that this happened two years later; that it recommended the use of short-life housing for homeless families and that housing in redevelopment areas was opened up and subsequently used for this purpose.

In assessing the value of SCP work in this matter, we may say that Project studies and reports:

led to action on the part of agency staff. For instance, the senior social worker in the homeless family block examined the possibility of undertaking a study of factors affecting the housing of residents. The adviser for this service started her own surveys in relation to poverty;
helped to disrupt the normally controlled information flow by assisting service workers to penetrate beyong the public relations image behind which they sometimes shielded;
encouraged action and initiative from different levels in agencies. People at the top of the management structure were often badly informed of what was happening at the bottom, and vice versa. Often councillors were ill-informed about what chief officers were doing. Reports were used by workers to promote information and initiate debate on issues in their agencies;
changed the awareness of some service staff about their role in planning and assessment;
provided information to residents and agencies about needs in

the locality as well as service provisions pertaining to those needs.

2 *Secondment.* A social services worker was seconded to the Project for four months. This worker helped the area team from which he came to acquire a better understanding of the work of the Project; and he was able to use Project material to assist the team in becoming area orientated. In addition, his work led to meetings between the area team and local tenants' associations about neighbourhood issues.

3 *Advice centre.* The seconded worker was also instrumental in persuading his area team to open a Monday night advice centre at the Project office. This was staffed by social workers from the team.

4 *Development of community work.* The work of the Project had some impact on the development of community work within the social services department. At a meeting with service workers to review the Project's work, one local authority worker said the Project had given 'a big push' to the development of community work in the borough. SCP staff were also sought by local authority and voluntary community workers for consultation and support.

5 *Models in SCP practice.* Many workers saw the Project as a model and some elements of its practice were reproduced elsewhere. For instance, a multi-service group was started in north Lambeth by a settlement community worker.

6 *Case referral.* Neighbourhood groups revealed new work for services. The referral network was also strengthened by increases in knowledge between agency staff in north-west Southwark. As relationships developed, staff were better able to identify reciprocal interests and they became more prepared to refer clients to other services. This had negative as well as positive consequences for clients, some of whom have traditionally been able to benefit from fragmented and isolated service systems. The unity achieved between agency staff strengthened service operations and hence a worker's capacity to resist exploitation by clients.

7 *The Multi-Service Group.* The work of the Group has already

been discussed and we must take into account the following considerations in assessing its value:

agency workers have acquired more knowledge of needs and services in the locality by attending the Group;
communication between residents and services has been fostered in the Group. Awareness has developed of the need for local participation in order to tackle problems more effectively, while local people have become more aware of the complexities of services operating in the area;
joint studies and reports have increased information available to service workers and residents and some local action has resulted;
some new services have developed locally such as an advice centre, an extra playgroup, and an evening meeting place for residents;
there has been more open and honest acknowledgement of unmet need among services represented on the Group;
the Group has served as a model for those concerned with the implementation of the Seebohm report's findings. The Group has also been regarded as an exciting experiment by people learning about or professionally responsible for social planning;
the proposal from the Group for a multi-service centre on the estate illustrated a new willingness on the part of agency staff to achieve more integrated services. Representatives from the Group joined officials from the Town Hall to work on the proposal for the centre. This representation included the local tenants' association and adventure playground committee.

8 *The Southwark Playground Association.* A Project worker played an important part in the development of this association, which was concerned with co-ordinating interest in, and the promotion of, play facilities in the borough.

4 THE SITUATION AFTER THE WITHDRAWAL OF THE SCP

An important part of the assessment of a community work project is to consider what it 'left behind' after its withdrawal. This section briefly indicates some of the major areas in which local residents in north-west Southwark continue to engage in community activities.

Southwark North Action Groups

The Southwark Community Project did not necessarily expect to leave behind a locally-managed community work base after its withdrawal. There was, however, a commitment to withdrawing with the least possible disruption to the neighbourhood. This commitment could have been implemented differently by the groups. It might have meant, for instance, linking tenants' associations with other support facilities in the neighbourhood or ensuring that playgrounds had an adequate knowledge base for fund raising or helping the North Southwark Community Development Group raise money to employ its own workers.

By January 1972, the Project workers began to make it known that 1972 would be the last year of the Project's operations. Likewise, it was decided to take no students from the National Institute for the 1972–3 academic year. December 1972 was set as a possible date for withdrawal with the expectation that Project workers would spend some six months preparing a written account of their work. There was, in fact, little response by groups to these notices of the imminence of the Project's withdrawal, but by April 1972 discussions were initiated about what would happen when the Project left.

By the end of May, these discussions became more formally organised and a working party was set up to explore possibilities. Withdrawal was also discussed at team meetings and meetings with users. The working party considered a number of options for action after withdrawal, and, in the event, it decided to raise funds in order to employ a community worker and to maintain a locally-managed community work base. The weeks between this decision and the summer of 1972 were full of hard work and anguish for users as they attempted to form themselves into a viable federation of neighbourhood groups. It was decided to exclude service agencies from the federation which became known as the Consortium of the Users of the Southwark Community Project; it was also decided to ask for funding for three community workers and secretarial support, although some people argued that a more viable proposal would be for one worker with supporting services.

The Consortium's fund-raising appeals were unsuccessful. One problem for the users was the difficulty of registering as a charity. However, sufficient money was raised locally to cover the first year's running costs and premises in the area were obtained from Peabody Housing Trust for a peppercorn rent. The National Institute granted the Consortium £1,800 to employ its own worker and arranged for the installation of services and telephones in the new premises.

The Consortium advertised for a community worker and an appointment was made to start in October 1972. The worker's brief included working with neighbourhood groups, supporting the work and development of the Consortium, and helping the Consortium raise long-term funding. The worker sought to inject purpose into the aims of the Consortium and to help formulate community action objectives that were more precise. It was with this consideration in mind that the name 'Consortium' was dropped and replaced by 'Southwark North Action Groups', a name that aggravated the difficulties of registration with the Charity Commissioners.

Southwark North Action Groups (SNAG) soon experienced its first major crisis – the newly appointed worker resigned and left in December. A second worker was appointed and began work in March 1972, only to resign two months later, inflicting doubts amongst SNAG members about their ability to manage the organisation. Another worker was subsequently appointed.

The situation of SNAG in December 1973 was as follows:

SNAG was managing and maintaining a community work centre in north-west Southwark that was used by a variety of local groups;

the centre was staffed by a part-time secretary and a full-time community worker; funds for the worker were to expire in April 1974;

the community worker was engaged in strengthening the management structure of SNAG and new groups had recently joined;

one trust had provided finance for part-time secretarial help and another had given SNAG a donation of £1,000 together with £480 a year for the next four years.

North Southwark Community Development Group

The tract of Southwark riverside between Blackfriars Bridge and Tower Bridge is considered by property developers and the local authority to be the most exciting opportunity for comprehensive redevelopment in London since the Great Fire. Since 1971 many speculative schemes have been produced for renewal; the local authority has prepared a strategy plan for the area and both have negotiated with one another at weekly meetings to hammer out an acceptable redevelopment scheme for offices, hotels, luxury flats and social amenities.

The North Southwark Community Development Group (NSCDG) was formed in May 1972 as an association of neighbourhood groups and service agencies concerned with north Southwark. The Group set itself the task of studying the development plans and the plan of the local authority and detailed criticisms of these plans were subsequently produced. The Group pressed for redevelopment in north Southwark that met the needs of local and borough residents for jobs, better homes, play-space, and better services and transport which did not violate the historical heritage of the Southwark riverside.

The work of the Group caught the attention of the London Organisation for Student Community Action which gave it £1,300 to employ its own research worker. In October 1973, the Group successfully applied under the Urban Aid programme for money to operate a community planning centre in north Southwark and £6,000 per annum has been allocated for the next five years.

The Playgrounds

The two committees concerned with playground provision achieved their aims of opening adventure playgrounds in their neighbourhoods. Following their hard work and successful fund raising, Mint Street acquired a site and employed play leaders paid by the Inner London Education Authority. They were also successful in acquiring funds from the Urban Aid programme. They are now developing a site for under-fives play provision and are hoping to employ a worker. They have also opened club facilities for older teenagers and wish to raise funds to employ a youth club leader. The committee is playing an important part in representing the rights and interests of young people in the area in their negotiations with the police, employers and others. Likewise, the Rockingham Adventure Playground Association manages an adventure playground on the estate and has acquired an Urban Aid grant to improve the site and employ a play leader.

On the service side, the Multi-Service Group continues to meet, and the weekly advice centre provided by the social services area team still operates from the offices of Southwark North Action Groups. Work is well in hand in planning the multi-service centre and the construction of the community hall on the Rockingham estate.

CONCLUSION

This assessment of the work of SCP indicates the potential of a coalition of neighbourhood groups and one kind of community work resource for effecting major changes in a locality. The demolition of tenements and the rehousing of over a thousand families, the provision of play facilities and the number of other changes that have been described in this book seem to confirm the potency of the coalition and the contribution made by the Southwark Community Project to improving the well-being of those in north-west Southwark.

The contribution of the Southwark Community Project was achieved on limited funds and staff resources within three and a half years. How much more might we expect from substantial and consistent action over longer periods and at many different levels in areas like north-west Southwark?

Chapter 10

CONCLUSION: SOME ISSUES AND PROBLEMS

In this chapter we examine some of the issues that have emerged in our discussion of community work practice in the Southwark Community Project. We shall look at two major areas of interest. First, we shall investigate more thoroughly some of the notions about resources with which we began the book. Second, we shall look at the question of coalitions and contracts.

1 NEIGHBOURHOOD RESOURCES

Efforts at community change of the kind described in previous chapters are mostly concerned with influencing particular kinds of tangible and intangible resources. The former would include, but would not be limited to, many of the resources already referred to – new housing, playspace, better maintenance services, and so forth. This category of tangible resources would be equivalent to the three resource categories identified in the first chapter, namely *material*, *service* and *organisational support* resources. Within the category of intangible resources we refer to attitude changes in the officials who work in the service agencies concerned with allocating and distributing material and organisational support services. If the change is successful, these officials become 'more sympathetic', 'more community-orientated', 'more flexible', and 'more enlightened' in the use of their discretionary powers. We also refer in this category to the attempts mostly associated with minority or stagmatised groups to enhance some parts of their stock of what we referred to in Chapter 1 as 'internal support resources'. Such groups often seek, or acquire as a spin-off, improvements in their self-respect, self-image and significance within the wider community. Finally, the category of intangible resources refers to the acquisition by local people of the kind of organisational knowledge and skills described in earlier chapters.

Transactions about resources occur between resource demanders and resource holders. Transactions of these kinds, where people identify their needs and take collective action in respect of them, are commonly referred to in community work practice and literature as 'redistributing resources', albeit at a local or borough level. Community work stresses the potency of material resources external to a local group, and the potential of intangible resources (e.g. indigenous leadership, collective identity, organisational skills, etc.) within the group to increase the material resources that it needs. The primary feature of this model of transaction which emphasises the potential of indigenous resources to redistribute material resources is shown in Figure 10.1 where housing is used as an example.

Housing estate   Housing department

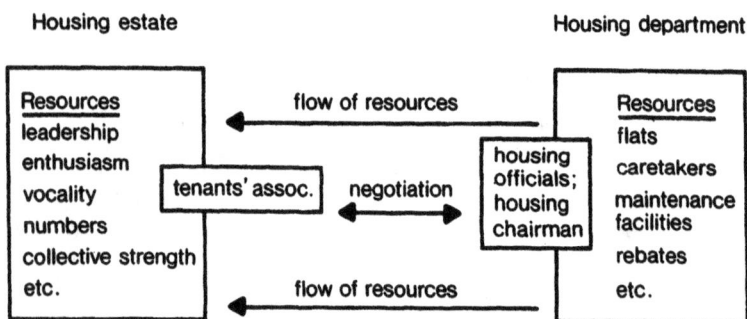

Resources | flow of resources | Resources
leadership | | flats
enthusiasm | | caretakers
vocality | tenants' assoc. | negotiation | housing officials; housing chairman | maintenance facilities
numbers | |
collective strength | | rebates
etc. | flow of resources | etc.

To look at community action from this perspective is helpful. But the variety of transactions described in preceding chapters between local groups and resource holders leads us to believe that the reality is more complex than a simple linear flow from resource holders to resource demanders. The work of the Southwark Community Project indicates, first, that the notion of resource redistribution/acquisition is imperfect because it obscures the diversity of ways in which community groups wish to influence decision-makers about resources. And, second, the flow is often two-way: the target[1] of the change effort may be as much a recipient of benefits from local groups as a provider of resources to them. We discuss each of these issues separately.

Resource transactions

Table 10.1 is a matrix that indicates, on the top horizontal line, six primary types of transactions about resources that we have

[1] The term 'target' in this chapter refers to those people and agencies that the community worker or neighbourhood group needs to change or influence in order to achieve their objectives.

identified in the work of the SCP. The left-hand vertical column lists some of the functional fields in which community workers and community groups traditionally operate.

resource acquisition

where community groups achieve an increase in or an addition to a stock of particular resources, both tangible and intangible. The group and its constituency acquires resources to which it has previously had little or no access. The acquisition of new housing by the tenants' associations in north-west Southwark is a good example.

resource rejection

where residents or a group oppose and reject the proposed introduction of resources to their community. The most striking example of resource rejection in north-west Southwark is found in the attempts of the North Southwark Community Development Group to keep hotel, office and commercial redevelopment out of their community. Examples are provided from other areas by airport and motorway opposition groups. The opposition of inner-city working-class groups to luxury flat developments also counts as resource rejection.

resource administration

where local residents or a community group take on responsibility for administering and managing a local resource (such as a playground, or short-life housing) but where the resources are owned and/or financed by, for instance, the local authority.

resource provision (self-help)

where residents attempt to provide services outside and independently of the formal structure of service provision.

resource improvement

where groups make an improvement in the quality of existing resources and services.

resource conservation

where groups attempt to conserve existing resources in the face of a threat to remove or reduce them. Thus one group may want to conserve an historic building or an open space whilst another may want to conserve the real incomes of the members in the face of impending rent increases. Community groups who help local people to resist evictions or harrassment by landlords are engaged in the conservation of a housing resource.

The boundaries of these transactions are not always certain or clear, and there may be difficulty in deciding in which category a transaction is to be placed. For instance, the efforts of Chaucer House Tenants' Association to achieve rehousing for its constituents may be seen either as a resource rejection or, if we look at it from the perspective of the tenants, as resource acquisition (new homes). Likewise, the efforts of Mint Street mothers to open and manage a playground may be seen both as resource acquisition and resource administration. Again, success in modifying the views of officials in the local offices of the Department of Health and Social Security in regard to stigmatized groups (i.e. resource improvement) may lead to greater use of discretionary powers and hence to increased welfare benefits (i.e. resource acquisition).

There are many benefits gained from examining the material in this book with this framework of resource transactions.

First, it may help us better to conceptualise the development of a community group through several kinds of transactions about resources. For instance, we can plot the progress of housing groups who often start with an interest in improving maintenance facilities on an estate and move on to other kinds of transactions like resisting evictions and rent increases.

Second, the framework enables us to categorise and describe the varied number of transactions (i.e. 'community issues') with which a group might be concerned. Table 10.2 indicates the number of transactions with which Chaucer House Tenants' Association was concerned. The tenants' association was first interested in cosmetic improvements in the block but moved on to negotiate with the local authority for demolition of the slum and rehousing of families. After several years of conflict with the authority, the block was demolished and a new policy announced to rehouse all further homeless families directly into the main housing pool. Table 10.2 shows how varied were the interests of the tenants' association. The problem such diversification posed for the community worker was that many of these transactions strained against the association's primary objective of 'breaking-up' the community in the block and dispersing residents to adequate housing. The complexity of the tenants' association's transactions points again to the tensions and contradictions that may exist

Table 10.1 TYPES OF RESOURCE TRANSACTIONS IN SEVERAL AREAS OF SERVICE

	Resource acquisition	Resource rejection	Resource administration	Resource provision (self-help)	Resource improvement	Resource conservation
Claimed Income	welfare rights and benefits			alternative publicity service; growing and distributing food co-operatively	more responsive officials; more humane treatment of stigmatized groups	opposing cuts in benefits
Housing	slum-clearance and rehousing; squatting	opposing developments of luxury flats	squatting – acting as a 'housing authority' in distributing tenants amongst empty properties given to the squatters by the local authority		improving maintenance facilities	resisting evictions; resisting rent increases
Environment		opposing the introduction of motorways; airports; office redevelopment			cosmetic neighbourhood improvements	opposing demolition of historic buildings
Play	more play facilities		parent-managed playgrounds; management of facilities by others (e.g. the local authority)	volunteer-run playgrounds; parents raising money and acting as playleaders	transforming static into adventure playgrounds	preventing the redevelopment of open space for commercial uses

Table 10.2 RESOURCE TRANSACTIONS OF CHAUCER HOUSE TENANTS' ASSOCIATION

Chaucer House TA	Resource acquisition	Resource rejection	Resource administration	Resource provision	Resource improvement	Resource conservation
housing	to close the block and rehouse tenants				maintenance, caretaking facilities	resisted evictions from the block
under-fives provision					investigated the under-use of a neighbouring playgroup	
work with services and other agencies	helped to open up a local weekly advice surgery provided by the social services department					helped tenants preserve their rights in the face of police action
youth facilities				opened youth club in empty flat; Xmas parties and trips to seaside		
grant-income				gave money to tenants in a crisis		

	Resource acquisition	Resource rejection	Resource administration	Resource provision (self-help)	Resource improvement	Resource conservation
claimed income	helped to form a local claimants' union				succeeded in getting the Dept. of Health and Social Security to send tenants' benefits to their flats rather than to the welfare office	helped tenants resist threatened cuts in benefits

between the objectives of a neighbourhood group. Apart from the tensions between collective objectives, individuals or minorities within a group may emphasise different objectives, and there may be yet other concerns among the broader population that the community group represents.

Third, different kinds of human resources may be better suited to some kinds of transactions than to others. For instance, residents who work effectively in a community group concerned with resource improvement or administration may not work as effectively with transactions about resource acquisition and vice versa; many of the local residents who successfully fought to acquire the Mint Street playground site were not as interested and effective in resource administration.

Fourth, the framework helps to identify some of the knowledge that community workers may require to work with groups engaged in a variety of resource transactions. Community workers who have experience and skills in resource acquisition and rejection may have neither the interest nor expertise to offer to groups concerned with transactions about resource improvement or administration. This has implications for community work training that mirrors some of the current discussions about the teaching of casework, group work and community work in social work courses. Do community work courses seek to turn out workers skilled in working in-depth with one or two types of resource transactions; or do they want to produce workers who can intervene effectively along the whole range of transactions that we find in community activities?

Mutuality and Difference in Resource Transactions

Community work traditionally emphasises the one-way flow of resources from resource holders and service providers to community groups and their constituents. We tend to think primarily of the new resources and improved services and more sympathetic and caring attitudes of bureaucratic officials that are the consequences of the intervention of a community group. But agencies that provide services also benefit as a result of their transactions with community groups. This mutuality of benefit is often overlooked or thought unimportant as agencies struggle to respond to the change proposals of community groups. Agencies will be too painfully aware of negative factors like hostile exposure by the media, irritated councillors, and inter-agency tensions.

Service agencies may even face a reduction in their stock of resources as a result of their transactions with groups; for instance, where groups implement rent strikes, resist rent increases and evictions, and seek to preserve an open site for play purposes rather than office development that would increase the local authority's rate returns. The resource conservation of community groups may be, from the service provider's point of view, tantamount to resource deprivation.

On the other hand, agencies will acquire positive benefits from their transactions with local groups. The awareness of agency personnel of these benefits, the value attached to them and their expected predominance over negative factors will help to determine the response of an agency to a group's demands. What are these benefits?

First, it is important to recognise the interdependence of the action and the target system within the change effort. For example, an agency that is the target of change for an action group composed of tenants can provide certain resources without which the desired change could not take place. If we take the example of a tenants' association seeking to have a slum demolished, the housing authority is not only the target system (i.e. getting it to agree to demolition) but it also provides essential skills and resources without which the association's change proposal could not be implemented; new flats; removal expenses; expertise in rehousing and matching household needs to available types of flat; powers to compulsory purchase; and the capacity through rent rebates to help families cope with the higher rent of the new flats. Although the phase of negotiation between the action group and its target may be characterised by conflict, once the sought-after policy decisions have been achieved the action group is highly dependent on the resources and good-will of the target. To this extent, sub-systems within the action and target systems overlap. Policy-makers within the housing authority may remain part of the target system but their colleagues and subordinates in administrative positions comprise a sub-system that overlaps the action group.

Depending on the nature and timing of their response to a change proposal, agencies will acquire benefits from many transactions with community groups like laudatory press coverage, increased prestige within the complex of local authority departments and, important for elected representatives, the goodwill and (possibly) the votes of residents in the community who are favourably impressed by the agency's response to a neighbourhood change proposal. If a local authority acquires a reputation for constructive responses to such proposals, all kinds of finance and ideas may flow into its area from people and organisations wishing to innovate and experiment in community-based and community-spirited activities. The most durable benefit may be improvements in the efficiency of the agency and in its service provision. Resource transactions between an agency and a community group may precipitate changes, for instance, in the agency's practice and procedures, in its relationships with other agencies and in its ability to identify the particular strengths and weaknesses of agency personnel. It is an ironic consequence of community action that it helps in the renewal and strengthening of its target systems.

The mutuality of resource transactions can be seen more clearly when we take specific examples. First, a local authority that agrees to the requests of local residents to preserve a patch of ground for play purposes acquires management and administrative resources when the residents take on responsibility for managing the playground and employing play leaders. It benefits, too, if calls on its other resources (such as its maintenance department) are reduced because the playground results in a fall-off in vandalism on council property in the neighbourhood. In a similar way, its social work resources and the efforts of the police and the probation service may be redeployed if the playground leads to reduced delinquency rates and the better take-up of other resources for young people like the schools, swimming pools, and evening classes.

Second, a group that seeks to oppose a planning application for an office development may be seen as allies by local authority planners who are hostile to, or undecided about, the merits of the application. Local opposition may strengthen the case for refusal, particularly if the matter goes to public inquiry.

The mutuality of benefit from many resource transactions is linked to a point made in the introduction to Chapter 4. We stated that there was relatively little difficulty for the worker in making contact with his peers in other professions and services. Although it may be relatively straightforward to make such contacts we must not gloss over the real difficulties of getting into a working relationship with service professionals. We found, for instance, that workers without social work training or other professional background were disadvantaged in their work with professionals in the social services comrpared to colleagues who could establish their credentials in, for instance, casework or other local authority service. There is also the difficulty in the reverse situation of being accepted in a 'community work role' if one was previously of the same profession as the other person.

A primary difficulty for many community workers intending to work with service agencies rather than neighbourhood groups is that of defining the community work function, and the necessity for it, in terms that help service personnel to accept it as a useful contribution to social services. Service personnel would ask 'How can the Project help?'; 'What am I, my agency and its clients, likely to gain from collaborating with this outside agency, the Southwark Community Project?' They were understandably ambivalent about working with Project staff if they anticipated that collaboration would lead to exposing the failures of service provisions or if they were not clear about the benefits that would come from co-operating with the Project and other agencies.

We have already alluded in Chapter 3 in the section on the 'Dual Approach' to some of the ways in which the Project's involvement with neighbourhood groups reduced the capacity of Project staff to build instrumental relationships with service agencies. Another dimension to this issue is that service personnel were initially very hesitant to give information about services (including their functions) when they knew that the information might be made available to neighbourhood groups using the Project. In situations where residents and service personnel came together to review service-delivery problems (e.g. the Multi-Service Group) it became an important task for the community worker to achieve recognition of the mutuality of the benefits likely to be gained from such joint efforts.

2   COALITION AND CONTRACT

Chapters 5, 6 and 7 described the interaction of neighbourhood groups and the Southwark Community Project as a 'coalition'. Each party to the coalition contributed skills and resources without which their individual and shared goals seemed less likely to be achieved.

We conventionally think that coalitions are formed by parties which have a developed sense of identity and destiny, a functioning organisational structure and tested rules and procedures for decision-making. Our use of the term 'coalition' in a community work setting is at odds with this conventional usage to the extent that the above conditions were often absent. We noted in earlier chapters, for example, that it is part of the community worker's task to help to create the other side of the coalition; that it is part of his work to enable neighbourhood groups to develop a sense of identity, an organisational structure and procedure for decision-making.

We might look for the consensual elements of this coalition – the record of what has been agreed upon by the parties in the change effort – in the contract established between worker and neighbourhood groups. Pincus and Minahan[1] have identified three fundamental elements agreed upon in social work contracts:

the major goals of the parties;
the tasks to be performed by each party to achieve the goals;
the operating procedures for the change process.

In the next section we examine the factors that seem to facilitate and constrain contract-making in community work.

Opening Moves

In Chapter 4 we indicated many of the ways in which community workers make contact with residents who may be motivated to join in collective action about local issues. The community worker has a mandate from his agency to identify and make contact with local residents. In this situation, residents are *potential* clients of the community work agency, or *potential* partners in an enterprise to effect change. Once contact has been made, the worker has then to influence and motivate residents to take part in a collective change effort, to become *actual* partners in the enterprise. We saw in Chapter 4 how often the worker seeks out residents who have a strong motivation to participate in collective action.

Unlike other branches of social work, community work relies exclusively on residents who participate voluntarily in interaction with the worker. There is no referral system in community work, as we understand it from casework; nor are there statutory responsibilities for community work. Thus, we could expect that those who

---

[1] A. Pincus and A. Minahan, *Social Work Practice: Model and Method* (Peacock Publishers, Illinois 1973), p. 164.

commit themselves to active membership in a community organisation are well motivated by virtue of their voluntary participation, and the extent to which they are affected by the local problem about which they seek change.

The Major Goals of the Parties

The community worker has a major responsibility to help the group define its primary problem and thus the goals that confront it as it sets about negotiations with decision-makers. Often residents will form a group and enter into a relationship with the community worker with little understanding of specific goals. 'Let's get together to do something about the estate', may be the sentiment which precipitates group formation. It is the task of the nascent group and the worker to spell out more precise goals in the change effort. It is at this stage that the worker will have to explain what *his* goals are – he will be expected to say why he is there, why he (perhaps a stranger from outside the community) has a stake in the resolution of a particular neighbourhood grievance. 'What's in it for him?' residents will ask themselves.

There are a number of factors that will determine the success with which the worker answers these queries and hence is able to fashion a meaningful contract. The first is the extent to which residents understand the community worker's role. We have already noted that residents are unlikely to have a clear notion of what exactly the worker will contribute to the coalition. It is our experience that workers cope with this problem uneasily; they themselves may have doubts about the ethics of intervening to help people organise; they may dismiss the notion of a 'contract' as so much social work nonsense and assert that what matters is their sense of identity with, and commitment to, the neighbourhood which recognises them as reliable, trustworthy helpers. It is not difficult for workers to take up this last position: we saw in Chapter 6 the importance of expressive values in the relationships that developed between SCP workers and leading members of neighbourhood groups.

The second factor is the immediacy and pressing nature of the issues confronting the nascent group. It is extremely tempting for both worker and group to be content with a vaguely worded declaration of the worker's intent to help. For example, we find that one worker said of himself:

'I introduced myself as from the SCP where we were concerned to help people with any problems or difficulties that they may face . . . I made it clear that we did not help people as individuals but as groups, for instance, tenants' associations, and I gave them some local examples of our work.'

This kind of statement may achieve an entrée for the worker but it does little to formulate the ingredients of a contract.

A third factor is the worker's inability always to be explicit about his major goals. It would be a foolhardy worker, for instance, who spelt out for a group that he would help them with their organisational needs, as we have defined these in Chapter 6.

A major difficulty for the worker in formulating a contract is that goals change and are modified in the light of group experience. Each goal change of this kind would indicate that ongoing renegotiation of the contract between worker and group is necessary. But there is little evidence from the records of workers at the SCP that their contracts were reviewed as groups redefined their interests. Workers presented blank cheques to groups: 'Here I am, use me and my project's resources as you will.' The workers drift with this relationship as the group moves from goal to goal. This is in contrast to an alternative form of contract-making where the worker might say: 'I shall help you organise yourselves as a tenants' association. When you have organised, we can then review the situation to see the ways, if any, in which I can help you meet your objectives.' Partialising goals in this way provides effective contracts through which the group may better understand the contribution of the worker, and through which the worker may strengthen the autonomy of the group and its capacity to decide whether or not it needs him. All too often workers and groups assume that the worker's success in making contact with the residents and helping them organise into a group creates an inviolate niche for the worker which he occupies for the duration of the change effort.

Tasks to be Performed for Goal Achievement

In addition to helping to specify tasks the worker must also take responsibility for assessing the resources within the coalition that are relevant to task performance. Community workers refer more to 'tactics and strategies' than to 'tasks'. There is little evidence from SCP records that groups worked out their strategies to achieve change; groups tended to respond to events and crises as they occurred, living from one set of tactics to another. It is unlikely that many community workers would see agreement on tasks as a necessary ingredient in making a contract with a group. On the contrary, workers are likely to acquiesce in group decisions about tasks with which they disagree; they will accord self-determination a higher value, and allow the group 'to learn from its mistakes'.

Operating Procedures for the Change Process

The operating procedures with which SCP workers and neighbourhood groups ordered their interaction were rarely clarified by workers when they initiated work with groups. It was assumed, for instance, that groups could use the Project when they wished, that there would be no charge for most of the facilities, and that the worker would be available at all times. We noted in Chapter 5 that residents became dissatisfied with these procedures because of the great number of demands made upon the workers and other Project resources. It might have helped groups to accept the constraints on a worker's contribution to its work if workers had indicated to groups the nature of these constraints at 'contract-making sessions'.

Neither was there clarification of whether the worker could have direct access to members of the constituency that had elected the committee with which the worker co-operated; or of the terms under which the worker could discuss the work of the group at Project meetings; or the use to which the records of the worker could be put. In short, there was as little commitment to identifying and agreeing upon operational procedures as to making contracts about goals and tasks.

It is difficult to resist the conclusion that the coalitions that we have described in this book were based at best on contracts that were often assumed and not articulated and at worst on the personal identification and commitment of the workers; and on the dependence of the residents. However, there are other factors to consider. There may be features of community work that exacerbate the difficulties of establishing a contract between a neighbourhood group and a community worker. A group which is at an early, uncertain period of its life may be unable or unwilling to be specific about goals and tasks, and unsure of the ways in which the community worker can help in the change effort. It would be of no avail for a worker to push a group to articulate a contract if this resulted in the weakening or dissolution of the group or a lowering of morale amongst its members. A group may become alienated from the worker and the change effort if its difficulties in establishing a contract compound, or are compounded by, the difficulties in communication, values and attitudes that often occur between working-class people and middle-class community workers. In addition, the difficulties may lead to a contract that is differently understood by worker and group, and by different members of the group. Neither will the worker have any confidence that the group will accurately communicate the contract to its constituent members.

These are some of the issues a worker must consider in deciding on the degree of specificity and deliberateness of contract that is feasible and/or desirable. He might also consider the confusion for local people of his having contracts with more than one group in the same area, particularly where there is overlapping membership among groups. He would also face difficulties in 'renegotiating' contracts in the changing circumstances of the group's development. Who, for instance, is to decide the point at which contract changes are to be 'negotiated'? Transitions from one phase to another in a group's life are often accompanied by internal crises about leadership, trust, confidence and so forth. The worker would have to be certain that by introducing the issue of 'renegotiation' of contract he was not hindering the group in its transition.

Contracts in social work are valuable to the extent that they enable the helper and the helped to achieve success (however that is mutually defined) in the change effort. Community workers must decide for every particular situation on the feasibility and value of verbal and explicit contracts. It may be that most contracts in community work will be created or confirmed implicitly, through action, behaviour, attitudes and performance. We noted in earlier chapters the ways in which workers at the SCP were tested out by members of neighbourhood groups. The notion of a contract offers, at the very least, the opportunity to community workers to make conscious appraisals and decisions about their interaction with a group through its different phases. This may inform the worker's contribution in ways not possible when he 'drifts' with the group from its inception to conclusion.

The development of a contract, with all that it entails in terms of specificity of goals and tasks, may also be a necessary precondition for effectively assessing the value of a particular worker's interventions with a group. Tangible products may indicate success and achievement in respect of the goals of a group or of a coalition or of a project; but they are no more than prima facie evidence that the interventions of an individual worker with a particular group have been effective.

In talking about the assessment of an individual piece of community work (rather than of a programme or project) we are really asking 'What was the relationship between the worker's intervention with "X" tenants' association and that association's development as a group and its success in achieving its goals?' The notion of a contract provides a base point from which we may be able:

to identify the goals that the worker sets for himself as a change agent;

to determine the appropriateness of these goals to the nature of the group, its perception of its primary problems and its definition of its major objectives;

to determine the appropriateness and efficacy of the tasks that the worker carries out in order to achieve his goals.

SUMMARY

Transactions about resources occur between neighbourhood groups and decision-makers; and within groups between the indigenous group members and the community worker.

The first kind of transactions are varied, ranging from resource acquisition to resource conservation. Distinguishing between the different kinds of transactions may help us better to understand the different skills and attributes required by both residents and workers in each kind of transaction.

The work of the Southwark Community Project indicated that it is not always feasible or appropriate to base the second kind of transaction – that between community worker and the group – upon well articulated contracts, with mutually agreed upon specificity about the goals and tasks of the worker and the group. We identified a 'drift' pattern for interventions – the worker gains an initial entrée to the group and drifts through the different phases of the group's activities and needs, creating and confirming contracts implicitly through, amongst other things, his attitudes and service to neighbourhood groups.

Where it is feasible and appropriate, specificity about goals and tasks may facilitate the task of assessing a community worker's contribution to the development of a neighbourhood organisation.

Appendix A

A GUIDE TO STAFF, NEIGHBOURHOOD GROUPS AND SERVICE AGENCIES

FIELD STAFF

John Rea Price, February 1968 to July 1969
Dorothy Runnicles, May 1968 to January 1973
Elizabeth Radford, September 1968 to September 1971
Harley Frank, September 1970 to June 1972
David Thomas, September 1971 to January 1973
Henrietta Branford, October 1972 to December 1972
David Jones, who prepared the proposal for the Project. He was the Director from its inception until 1973.

ADMINISTRATIVE STAFF

Mrs M. Aldridge
Mrs P. Barclay
Mrs E. Brazier
Mrs L. Brookman
Miss J. Letts

Miss M. Littlefield
Mrs L. Shemeld
Mrs V. Uffindell
Miss J. Vollmer

There were, as well, numbers of students at the Project for varying periods of time, both from the National Institute and other training institutions. There were, too, a number of people involved in research or the teaching and/or practice of social services, including community workers who worked at the Project on a two-days-a-week basis, mostly for a period of a year. Finally, several visiting American professors at the National Institute became involved with Project work on a consultancy basis.

NEIGHBOURHOOD GROUPS AND RESIDENTS

Tenants' Associations

The Project worked with thirteen tenants' associations, from estates of different sizes and ages. These were: Arcadia Buildings, the Aylesbury Estate, the Bankside, Barnaby Buildings, Chaucer House, Goodwin Buildings, Guinness Buildings, Lawson Estate, Meadow Row, Queens

Buildings, Red Cross Way, Rockingham Estate, and Winchester Buildings.

These are the tenants' associations with whom there was substantial work done by the Project. The issues with which they were concerned included the demolition of slums and the rehousing of tenants (six of the thirteen associations); improved maintenance and repair services; play and recreational facilities; vandalism to estates; the physical redevelopment of north-west Southwark; the provision of advice services; and an interest in meeting the needs of certain groups of tenants like the elderly and the handicapped. Of course, there were many more tenants' associations in other parts of Southwark with whom the Project worked for very time-limited specific purposes such as the exchange of information, or help given to carry out a survey.

It is important to stress that all these tenants' asociations, like other kinds of groups, varied in size, objectives, representatives, accountability to tenants, and success in achieving goals. It is also important to note that the level of activity, participation and vitality of these associations varied over time. These associations made varying uses of Project resources. In addition, these associations, like the groups discussed below, used not only SCP resources but also those of other professionals in the area such as community workers from the area team of the social services department, the clergy, and others who had expertise or relevant information.

Playgrounds

Mint Street Adventure Playground Association
Rockingham Adventure Playground Association

A Project worker was instrumental in assisting playgrounds in other parts of the borough through her work as secretary of the Southwark Adventure Playground Association.

Other Neighbourhood Groups and Interests

Southwark North Action Groups (Borough and District Neighbourhood Association)
The North Southwark Community Development Group
Southwark Health Action Group
Early Warning Systems for Preventing Homelessness Group
Southwark Bridge Road Pedestrian Crossing Group
All Saviours Gardens Residents Group
St Saviours Parents' Association
Southwark Bridge Road Library Petition
Elephant Mothers' Group

These groups were respectively concerned with maintaining a community work base after the withdrawal of the SCP; the physical redevelopment of the area; the level of health care in the neighbourhood; the detection and prevention of homelessness; better pedestrian crossing facilities; the preservation of a church garden as a public amenity; participation in discussions about the future of a local school; protesting against the proposed closure of the local library; and providing a mutual support group for local mothers with young children.

This work with neighbourhood groups, and that outlined below with service agencies, was undertaken during the three and a half years between April 1969, when the Project moved into its shop-front premises, and January 1973 when it withdrew completely from Southwark. It should be noted that this list does not include the wide range of contacts and work between Project staff and individuals in the area, including residents and workers in organisations like local schools, churches, settlements, business firms, and students. We should also recognise the diversity of work undertaken by students at the Project on issues such as homeless vagrants, pub facilities, and caretaking facilities in the neighbourhood. The 'students' were professional workers taking mid-career training at the National Institute. They presented themselves in the area as part-time Project workers, though not disguising that they were on a training course.

WORK WITH SERVICE AGENCIES

The Project worked with the welfare and children's departments and later with the social services department and with the departments of planning, housing and health. In addition, the Project workers co-operated with the Southwark Council of Social Services, the Citizens' Advice Bureau and a number of settlements located in the London Borough of Southwark. Work was also initiated with the Southwark Adventure Playground Association and the Rockingham Estate Multi-Service Group.

The Project and its workers also undertook some work with other agencies and interest groups within and outside the borough. The most important that we might mention include: the Social Workers' Lunch Club, the Community Workers' Group, the Seebohm Study and Action Group, the British Association of Social Workers, the Southwark Family Squatting Association, the Association of London Housing Estates; and a variety of services including the Educational Welfare Service, Probation Service, the Police, Bermondsey Service for the Disabled, the Youth Service, and Save the Children Fund. Here again, the degree of involvement and time varied from one group to another.

Appendix B

REPORTS FROM THE SOUTHWARK COMMUNITY PROJECT

The following are the reports which the Southwark Community Project produced, or helped to produce jointly with other agencies and neighbourhood groups. These papers are no longer available for distribution, but those marked with an asterisk are in the library of the National Institute for Social Work.

Studies of Residents' Views – on two council estates: the Sumner Estate, SCP, 1968; the Rockingham Estate, 1969.
A Playground Survey in Southwark, Southwark Council of Social Service and Southwark Playground Association, 1969.*
Profile on Services – the function and operation of twenty-one services locally provided on the Rockingham Estate, SCP, 1970.
A Report on a Survey of those of Pensionable Age in the Sumner Estate, SCP, 1970.
A Multi-Service Centre – a unified approach to service provision in north-west Southwark, SCP and others, 1970.
A Preliminary Plan for a Multi-Service Centre, SCP, 1970.
Report on Homeless Families in Southwark, SCP, 1970.*
Working Paper on Methods of Analysing Needs, SCP and the Department of Planning and Architecture, London Borough of Southwark, 1970.*
The Public House as an Information Resource to the Community Worker, SCP, 1970.
The Collection and Monitoring of Information in the Social Service Department, SCP, 1970.
The Information Givers, SCP, 1970.
The Development of the Rockingham Advice Centre, SCP, 1971.
A Preliminary Proposal for Economic Development in North Southwark, D. Coleman, 1971.
A Report of an Investigation in an Area of the London Borough of Southwark into the Needs of Under-Fives and their Mothers, SCP, 1972.*
A Report on the Level of Health Care in North-West Southwark, SCP, 1970.

Services for Handicapped Young People in Southwark, Multi-Service Group, 1972.*

Focus on the Senior Citizen: Information on the Benefits and Services for the Elderly in North-West Southwark, Multi-Service Group, 1972.

INDEX

Abbey ward 40
Adventure playgrounds (*see* Play provision)
Association of Community Workers 21
Association of Neighbourhood Councils
  Hornsey Plan 101–2

BBC (*see* Media)
Blackfriars Settlement 51, 53, 156
'The Block' 97–100
Borough and District Neighbourhood Association (*see* Southwark North Action Groups)

Case Con 150
Cathedral ward 37, 38, 40, 41, 66
Chaucer House 42, 73, 93, 97–100, 105, 157, 158
Chaucer House Tenants' Association 97–100, 105, 181
Chaucer ward 40
Child Poverty Action Group 150
Children and Young Persons Act 49
Chronically Sick and Disabled Persons Act 49
Church Army 41
Church Commissioners 41
City of London Corporation 38, 41
Coalition 89–90, 130, 133, 161, 174, 185–6, 189
Collective action
  Costs 102–6; Strength 94–106
Commercial service resources 29
Communication & Information Group 150
Communist Party 51
Community groups
  Administrative resources 132–3; Committees 163; Competition for resources 91–94; Contracts between worker and group 187– 91; Development phases 110–28; Finances 101, 117–19, 154, 171; Formation 74–88; Intervention phases 78–88, 109–29; Skills 28–9, 61, 96, 101, 114–17, 125, 160–64, 182; Steering groups 111–12; Strains of office 103–6; Strengths of collective action 94–106
Community resources 29–35, 40, 113–14, 121, 130–34, 150, 157–9, 175–85
  Value 31–5
Community work
  Aims 187–91; Time limit 108–9; Worker's opening moves 69–78, 82, 186; Worker's part in decision-making 122–9; Worker's role 107–29, 187–88
Consortium of the Users of the Southwark Community Project (afterwards 'Southwark North Action Groups') 171–2
Councillors (*see* Southwark, London Borough of)

Demonstrations (*see* Public meetings)

Environment, Department of 95
Evelina Children's Hospital 51

Goodwin Buildings 84, 157, 158
Greater London Council 39, 41, 44, 63, 65, 92, 96, 128
  Housing Department 44; Housing Study 1966 41
Guinness Buildings 157
Gulbenkian Report 21

Hays Wharf 43
Health & Social Security, Department of 25, 44, 104, 181
Homeless 20, 34, 42, 46, 47, 64, 73, 81, 92, 97–100, 122, 125, 168

For Product Safety Concerns and Information please contact our EU
representative GPSR@taylorandfrancis.com
Taylor & Francis Verlag GmbH, Kaufingerstraße 24, 80331 München, Germany

www.ingramcontent.com/pod-product-compliance
Lightning Source LLC
Chambersburg PA
CBHW050444280326
41932CB00013BA/2232

*9 7 8 1 0 3 2 0 4 3 0 4 3 *